The Politics of Birth

Dedication

For my daughter Tess, who keeps me going – with admiration for her wisdom, her understanding of the politics of birth and her many talents.

For Elsevier:

Commissioning Editor: Mary Seager
Development Editor: Rebecca Nelemans
Production Manager: Yolanta Motylinska
Project Management and Typesetting: Helius
Cover design: Pete Wilder
Page design: Julian Howell

The Politics of Birth

Sheila Kitzinger

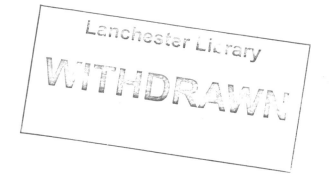

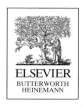

ELSEVIER
BUTTERWORTH
HEINEMANN

Edinburgh   London   New York   Oxford   Philadelphia   St Louis   Sydney   Toronto   2005

ELSEVIER
BUTTERWORTH
HEINEMANN

Cover design. Grateful acknowledgement to Rodney, Yvette and Kieran O'Dowd.

First published 2005
  Reprinted 2006

ISBN 0 7506 8876 9

British Library Cataloguing in Publication Data
A catalogue record for this book is available from the British Library

Library of Congress Cataloguing in Publication Data
A catalogue record for this book is available from the Library of Congress

Notice
Knowledge and best practice in this field are constantly changing. As new research and experience broaden our knowledge, changes in practice, treatment and drug therapy may become necessary or appropriate. Readers are advised to check the most current information provided (i) on procedures featured or (ii) by the manufacturer of each product to be administered, to verify the recommended dose or formula, the method and duration of administration, and contraindications. It is the responsibility of the practitioner, relying on experience and knowledge of the patient, to make diagnoses, to determine dosages and the best treatment for each individual patient, and to take all appropriate safety precautions. To the fullest extent of the law, neither the publisher nor the authors assumes any liability for any injury and/or damage.

The Publisher

ELSEVIER   your source for books,
journals and multimedia
in the health sciences

www.elsevierhealth.com

Working together to grow
libraries in developing countries
www.elsevier.com | www.bookaid.org | www.sabre.org
ELSEVIER   BOOK AID
International   Sabre Foundation

The
publisher's
policy is to use
**paper manufactured
from sustainable forests**

Printed in China

Contents

Preface

The idea for this book came from a regular Letter from Europe that I have written for the Blackwell Science publication *Birth: Issues in Perinatal Care* since the early 1990s, and these form the heart of some of the chapters. I am grateful to Blackwell Science (USA) for allowing me to incorporate them in the text. Other material is based on articles I have written for the *British Journal of Midwifery*, the *MIDIRS Digest* and *The Independent* and some passages in a book of mine, *Ourselves as Mothers*, which is now out of print, together with lectures I have given to midwives, sociologists, childbirth educators and birth campaigners around the world.

I want to thank the many women with whom I have discussed their experiences of birth and breastfeeding. I quote many of them and use some of their photographs. Thank you also, to the children who told me what it was like to be present at the births of siblings and drew pictures for me. I have learned a great deal from all the midwives, male as well as female, with whom I have discussed the issues addressed in these pages. My assistant, Emmeline Crause, was a tower of strength.

Sheila Kitzinger

Acknowledgements

For the photographs and other illustrations used in this book I want to thank the following people:

Anthea Sieveking, for generously giving her photograph of the Birthrights Rally (Ch. 6 and p. 50)

Beverley Lawrence Beech, for the photograph she took for Channel 4 of the prisoner in chains in the hospital (Ch. 20 and p. 186)

Caroline Flint and Francesca Hughes, for the happy photograph of a home birth (p. 143)

Catherine and Stephen Ream, for the beautiful pictures of their son's waterbirth 'This was so important to me! I lifted him up!' (Chs 11 and 22)

Uwe Kitzinger for the vivid photographs of Tess giving birth (Chs 1, 13, 14 and 15 and pp. 69, 94, 114, 118 and 127 and the photograph of Sheila dancing (p. 48)

Tess McKenney, for producing the photos in Chapters 3, 19, 21 and Useful Websites and Addresses and on pages 18, 24, 53 and 92. Also for the photographs of her giving birth (Chs 1, 13 and 14 and 15, and pp. 69, 94, 114, 118 and 127) and the photographs with her children (Ch. 5, and pp. 41 and 176)

Dickinson Healthcare Supplies for the photograph of a caesarean vacuum extraction (p. 37)

Gaumard Scientific, for the graphic photograph of the Maternal Simulator (p. 26)

Kedi Simpson, for the lovely photographs of her waterbirth, her children and their granny (Chs 2 and 12, and pp. 13 and 130)

Kirsten Millinson, for the tender photograph of her older children talking to the unborn baby (Ch. 8 and p. 71)

Michelle Fulcher, for the photo of the birth of a child – the birth of a father (Ch. 17)

Paul Beland, for the photograph of him with a gorgeous new baby (p. 145)

Yvette O'Dowd, for the dramatic pictures of her caesarean section (Chs 9 and 10, and pp. 38, 76 and 78)

Ricardo Jones MD, Brazilian Obstetrician, for the photograph of Nicole being supported in labour by her doula, Christina (Ch. 16)

Yehudi Gordon, for the drawing of episiotomy, taken from his chapter in the book of mine, *Episiotomy: Social and Emotional Aspects*, published by the National Childbirth Trust (p. 5)

Julia Harrison for the happy photograph of her and Tess breastfeeding in the garden (p. 41)

Sophie for her drawing of her spotty dog, Pongo, and her baby brother, in his mother's arms (Ch. 18 and p. 175)

The photograph in Chapter 21 is of a sculpture by Juliet Dyer.

I thank Roisin McAliskey for her perceptive and vivid description of being pregnant in prison (pp. 196–198).

I should also like to thank the following for permission to use excerpts from their own work:

Anne Enright (pp. 155–156)

Jennifer Worth (p. 167)

Lorna Davies (Table 12.1, pp. 108–109)

Penny Armstrong and Sheryl Feldman (pp. 11, 12, 69 and 70)

Tricia Anderson (Tables 15.1 and 15.2, pp. 148–151)

Dr Ian Young (pp. 138–139).

1
Giving birth

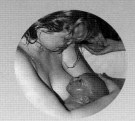

For human beings birth is never simply a matter of the shape of the pelvis and the size and presentation of the fetus. It is not just a biomechanical process. Like sex, it is to do with what is going on in our *minds*. The brain is the most important sexual organ. It is important in birth, too. This does not mean that all a woman need do is to have positive thoughts. Everything depends also on what is going on in the minds of those assisting the birth, the way it is conducted, and the relationships between all those involved. What we think and the connections made between ideas, everything we anticipate, what we hope for and fear – these are part of our birth culture.

Every society has its own birth culture. In northern industrial societies, and increasingly in the developing world, this is medical and technocratic.

Ritual guards the margins of life – the in-between states, the transition between different kinds of identity and the whole process of *becoming*. From being a child to being recognised as an adult, for example, is marked by puberty rites, and from being single to being married is characterised by wedding rites.

Ritual acts are symbolic. They represent another layer of meaning, and although they may appear to have a practical, even mundane, purpose, this is overlaid by symbolic significance. These symbols are not symbols in the individual unconscious, but are *shared* symbols in the culture and express social organisation and values. Birth and death – coming into life and leaving it – are surrounded by ritual in virtually every society. They are the greatest, and most universal, transitions of all and thus are heavily imbued with ritual.

Rites in a technocratic birth culture

Traditionally throughout the world, birth is a social process. It takes place in women's space, on female territory from which men are excluded. In sharing the rites of childbirth, women are bonded together in a nurturing act. They employ skills, including movement, massage, invocation and powerful imagery, that have been handed down from grandmothers through mothers and daughters. These unite them in empirical and esoteric knowledge. The conducted rites centre on the transformation of personal and social relationships, to make birth safe by creating social harmony and drawing on help from spiritual forces (represented by the gods and the ancestors), and expressing the dependence of human beings on the cosmic environment.

In northern industrial societies we have a technocratic birth culture. It is managed by professionals who depend on machines to read, diagnose and regulate everything that is done. It also employs ritual to make birth safe. But it is very different from traditional birth ceremonies. Ritual acts reinforce the power of the institution in which birth takes place and professional control over childbirth. They are used to de-sex birth and turn it into a medical process. Every intervention, including induction of labour, artificial stimulation of the uterus, episiotomy, instrumental delivery and caesarean section, can be used in a ritualised way if employed without discrimination and when not evidence-based.

Some rites with which most midwives will be familiar, such as the enema and shave, originated well before the introduction of modern birth technology. They have died out in many countries, to be replaced by new ceremonial acts, such as continuous electronic fetal monitoring.

Legitimisation of pregnancy

In a technocratic birth culture the first rite consists of the formal medical acknowledgement of pregnancy and classification of a woman as a patient. The doctor confirms that she is pregnant, assesses her risk status, fills in forms to register this, makes arrangements for the medical management of pregnancy, and books her into a hospital. She usually knew she was pregnant before this visit, but only now is the pregnancy legitimised.

The antenatal clinic

Complex ritual is used to regulate and de-sex pregnancy and birth and turn them into medical processes.

In all transitional rites, the ceremonial passage from one identity to the next is marked first by an act of separation. The initiate is set apart from peers and must attend a designated place where everything that is done is controlled by ritual.

If a pregnant woman does not attend clinic visits regularly she becomes a 'defaulter', and is perceived as failing in her duty to the fetus, rather like a soldier who is a deserter.

The ceremonial of the antenatal clinic and regular screening procedures, including fetal monitoring and ultrasound scans, serve as a rite of passage, symbolically registering the significance of the transition to birth for the society. Pregnancy is a medical process in which the fetus is a commodity that is monitored and its growth recorded and supervised. The mother is relevant only in so far as she is the container for the fetus. In fact, she is an obstacle to inspection of the fetus.

Ultrasound dating of pregnancy

In traditional birth cultures the expectant mother does not rely on any other authority to tell her when her baby is due. It is part of women's knowledge. Authoritative knowledge about pregnancy time, as with all other knowledge about birth, is not professional property. This knowledge is shared between women.

In a technocratic culture, in contrast, dimensions of pregnancy and birth time are defined by the obstetrician. A woman's own knowledge of when intercourse occurred and when she ovulated is deemed irrelevant. The only authoritative knowledge is specialised and dictated by an ultrasound scan in early pregnancy.

Depilation

The cutting of hair is a symbol of social control.[1] The novice monk's head is shaved, and when a man joins the army or becomes a prisoner his hair is cut close to his head. Shaving of the head is a symbol of mourning in many cultures. The shaving of a woman's pubic hair at the onset of labour was common in the UK until the 1980s. Her perineum was made as bald as a hard-boiled egg and her external sexual organs returned as far as possible to a pre-pubertal state. This is still done in many hospitals in the USA, Eastern Europe and developing countries. The practice started when poor women entering charity hospitals often had lice in their pubic hair. There was never any evidence that shaving reduced the number of bacteria on the perineum. In fact, research shows that infection is more likely when a razor has been used, since surface cells are scraped and allow the introduction of bacteria.[2]

Purging

The shave was followed by an enema, a ritual purging from pollution. We know now that it is not only uncomfortable, but unnecessary.[3] Yet the practice persists in ex-Communist countries and in many Eastern countries. It demonstrates to the patient that the territory of her body, including the functioning of its inner parts, is under the control of hospital staff.

Here is one doctor's description of medicalised birth rites in his own country, Taiwan:

> Taiwan has transformed itself from a developing to a developed country in recent decades ... In childbirth, medicalisation has taken hold throughout the

*obstetric profession ... On entering a delivery suite pregnant women undergo
a routine enema, routine pubic shaving, routine nil by mouth, routine
intravenous cannulation, and routine intravenous infusion ... Pregnant
women at term with rupture of the membranes before labour are subjected
to routine induction of labour. Expectant management for even the next
12–24 hours is perceived as too risky an alternative. Even pregnant women
at 36 weeks' gestation are subjected to the same routine protocol. All women
in labour undergo routine midline episiotomy.*[4]

Artificial rupture of the membranes

Routine ARM, still a standard practice in some hospitals, further reinforces the
woman's awareness of the obstetrician's control of her most intimate and
previously private body functions.

The tethered body

Most women are still put to bed in hospitals all over the world. Their movements
and the positions they adopt are strictly controlled. Electronic fetal monitoring
and an intravenous cannula further immobilise them, leaving them physically
helpless and trapped.

Research has shown that upright postures significantly reduce pain.[5] The supine
position can produce pressure on the inferior vena cava and the aorta and
interfere with oxygenation of the fetus. The lithotomy posture puts stress on
the maternal sacroiliac spine and on the perineum. But placing a woman in a
supine position and fixing her legs in lithotomy stirrups enables the caregivers
to control her in a way they cannot when she is free to move around.[6] Birth
then becomes like any other operation in which the patient is immobilised, and
power is unmistakably in the hands of the professionals. In most hospitals in
the USA women are still not allowed down off the delivery table.

The electronic monitor

The monitor tends to be used in a ritual way, too.[7] Even if it is not working
correctly, and if no one is analysing the print-out, caregivers believe it is
important. Obstetricians often say that this is because of anxiety about possible
litigation. Yet, even when this concern is not voiced, monitoring is like a St.
Christopher medal on a journey, a magic symbol to ensure safe passage through
dangerous territory.

Isolation and exposure of the genitals

When an obstetrician isolates and exposes a woman's vulva it becomes ritually
separate from that part of her body which she herself is allowed to control.
Transformed into a 'sterile field', it is out of bounds to her own touch. The sterile
field – not, in fact, sterile because of the juxtaposition of vagina and anus – is an
obstetric fiction by which a woman's genital area is depersonalised and de-sexed,

so that there is no longer a man looking at a woman's exposed vulva, but a doctor managing a patient.

Second stage ritual management

Management of the second stage of labour involves ritual commands either to push or to avoid pushing. It is difficult for caregivers to measure full dilatation with precision, but the fiction persists that if the cervix is assessed at 10 cm the woman should push, and if it is not yet 10 cm she must not. Authoritative judgement as to the appropriate time to push often runs counter to the mother's spontaneous impulses. In the absence of involuntary pushing urges she is ordered to take a deep breath, hold it, grasp her thighs, and push as hard and as long as she can. If she longs to push but the cervix is not considered adequately dilated, or if the designated authority – the obstetrician – is not available to licence her to push, she is told that she must resist the urge and pant and blow strenuously. These instructions, accompanied as they often are by threats that she will harm her baby or herself and by noisy concerted action to control her behaviour, impose both physiological and emotional stress, and may be part of a process that leads to instrumental delivery.[8, 9]

Episiotomy

If the woman has succeeded in achieving a vaginal birth, it may be completed by the final flourish of an episiotomy. Ceremonial mutilation takes place. Her sexual organs are surgically incised and then sutured.[6]

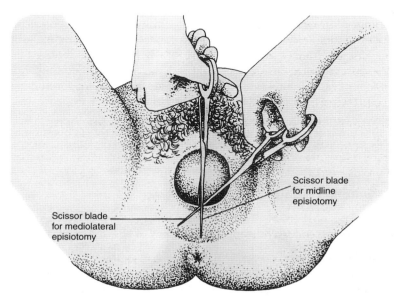

Scissor blade for midline episiotomy

Scissor blade for mediolateral episiotomy

Episiotomy became widespread, despite no research evidence of its benefits

Episiotomy became part of routine management in the USA in the 1920s and was taught to generations of medical students by Dr Joseph DeLee of Chicago. He believed that sedating the patient, slicing open her perineum between the vagina and the anus, and delivering by forceps, prevented babies turning into 'idiots and psychopaths', avoided prolapse of the uterus, slack pelvic floor muscles and vesicovaginal fistula, and was of benefit to marriages because 'virginal conditions are often restored'.[10]

American doctors advocated routine 'prophylactic' episiotomy (that is, whether or not there was any indication of stress on the perineum) and tight suturing well into the 1970s. Many still do so. They inserted what they often called 'the husband's stitch', an extra suture so that the male partner could derive sexual pleasure from a tightly gripping vagina. He would be grateful to the obstetrician who had made his wife 'as good as new' – that was the phrase used. Women were not consulted about this. And doctors did not realise that many sexual problems after childbirth were the direct result of episiotomy and suturing of the perineum.

Routine episiotomy soon became part of British obstetric and midwifery practice too. The rate shot up with the switch from home to hospital births. At one London hospital, the West Middlesex, until the domino scheme ('domiciliary in and out' – bringing a woman into hospital for delivery only) was introduced in 1971, community midwives assisting at home births had an episiotomy rate of 4%. When they went into hospital to do deliveries, it rose to 38% within 5 years.[11]

Right through the 1970s and 1980s midwives were made to feel deeply ashamed if a mother had a tear. It was a disgrace. No-one was ever criticised for an unnecessary episiotomy. But, to the credit of British midwives, as soon as the practice of routine episiotomy was challenged, rates went down dramatically – in some hospitals from over 70% to around 40% in a matter of weeks. At the John Radcliffe Hospital, Oxford, where the rate was near 70% in primiparas, the episiotomy rate plummeted by 38% for primiparas and 58% for multiparas between the years 1980 and 1984, most of this before research evidence was published.[11] Episiotomy rates in UK hospitals are now around 14%, but in some units are as high as 25%. Midwives have a powerful role in questioning unnecessary and possibly harmful interventions and building practice that is research-based and woman-centred.

Clock-watched labour

Time dominates birth in the 21st century. In studying the modern technology of childbirth it is easy to forget the oldest technology of all – the clock. Yet, as we shall see in Chapter 3, it is the basis of all the other technology and obstetric interventions that are employed. Clock-watching had become the norm in the technocratic birth culture of nearly all the northern industrial nations by the 1970s. The clock has had a tremendous impact on how labour is managed. It produces a profound effect, not only on a woman's experience of birth, and her sense of achievement or failure, but also dictates the midwife's role as manager and recorder of events in time, rather than as a skilled companion, who intervenes when there is evidence of undoubted benefit, but who otherwise has the confidence to observe and wait.[12]

What is 'normal' birth?

It is tempting to think of the technocratic model of birth as 'normal', and of all other birth cultures as aberrations from that norm. Yet if we look at birth from a global perspective throughout history and across cultures, it is this medicalised model that is strange. It is a culture of birth in which mothers, separated from women's network of loving support, deliver in an alien institution. A personal life transformation is under the control of people who are often strangers in a hospital, an institution which usually treats those who are ill or injured. It is birth in the absence of an intimate one-to-one continuing relationship between the midwife and the mother, in which a midwife's lasting relationship with the baby who is coming to birth and with the family – characteristic of traditional cultures – is usually absent.

In Europe and North America childbirth is undoubtedly safer than in the impoverished countries of the southern hemisphere. But in the process of making it safer it has been pathologised.

In the chapters that follow we shall explore in more detail how our birth culture operates, both for those who are employed within the field and for women for whose service it is intended, and the ways in which this affects behaviour and thinking.

References

1. Hallpike CR 1978 Psychological and sociogical theories of body symbolism. In: Polhemus T (ed) Social aspects of the human body. London: Penguin, p 145

2. Romney ML 1980 Pre-delivery shaving: an unjustified assault? Journal of Obstetrics and Gynaecology 1:33–35

3. Romney ML, Gordon H 1981 Is your enema really necessary? BMJ 282:1268–1271

4. Yeh PS 2002 Childbirth in Taiwan is certainly overmedicalised [letter]. BMJ 325:104

5. De Jong PR, Johanson RB, Boxen P, et al 1997 Randomised trial comparing the upright and supine positions for the second stage of labour. British Journal of Obstetrics and Gynaecology 104(5):567–571

6. Kitzinger S 2000 Rediscovering birth. London: Little Brown, p 169

7. Grant A 1989 Monitoring the fetus during labour. In: Chalmers I, Enkin M, Keirse MJNC (eds) Effective care in pregnancy and childbirth, vol 2. Oxford: Oxford University Press

8. Bergstrom L, Siedel J, Killman-Hull L, Roberts J 1997 'I gotta push. Please let me push!' Social interactions during the change from first to second stage labor. Birth 24:3

9.   Caldeyro-Barcia R 1979 The influence of maternal bearing-down efforts during second stage on fetal wellbeing. Birth 6:17–21

10. DeLee J 1920 The prophylactic forceps operation. Transactions of the American Gynecology Society 45

11. Graham I 1997 Episiotomy: challenging obstetric interventions. Oxford: Blackwell Science

12. Page LA 2000 The new midwifery: science and sensitivity in practice. London: Harcourt Publishers

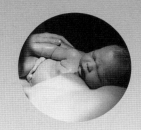

2
The birth place

In traditional cultures birth usually takes place in a small, private, dimly lit place where there are no intrusions, and where the woman can focus on and respond unselfconsciously to the physiological urges that impel her to adapt her breathing, posture, movements, and the sounds she makes, to the process of giving birth.

This may be in a secluded room in her own home or her mother's home, the local bathhouse that is used by women, a specially constructed seclusion hut, a hedged enclosure or a fern-bedded space on the forest floor.

Traditionally, when women have choice they give birth in an enclosed space like a nest, lined with moss, leaves, fur or soft fabric. Sometimes – as among the native Americans of the Great Plains – women give birth on a bed of sand, that can be swept up after the baby is born, or – as in Mexico – in a hammock that moulds itself to the shape of the mother's body.

The Kwakiutl of British Columbia used to line their shallow birth pits with soft cedar bark. Traditional societies continue in cultured form the biological process that other mammals and birds demonstrate when they select a secluded place and line their nests with soft hay or moss. In New Zealand the Maori birth hut was actually called 'the nesting house'.

In North America the colonists of New England prepared a 'borning room' in each white clapboard homestead. It was behind the central stove, would be comfortably warm, and the woman gave birth there against large feather pillows on a soft bed quilt.[1]

In Uganda the Baganda woman gives birth in the garden of her husband's mother's home, where she kneels grasping a tree, supported by a female member of her husband's family, while the midwife, who is one of her husband's relatives, kneels behind her ready to catch the baby.

The Manus of New Guinea give birth in special houses where the old women of the tribe live, built on stilts over the sea. In some Pacific Islands the mother went down to the margins of the sea, where she could immerse herself in the water after the birth, and in one Maori tribe she might give birth on the banks of a river that was sacred to her people.

In Sierra Leone birth often takes place in the club house of the Sande secret society, the organisation that educates women for adult roles and responsibilities, and the midwife is the *majo* or headwoman of the society. In some villages the Sande runs a dormitory-style house in which mothers stay with their babies until they have weaned them, often at about 18 months. The Sri Lankan woman gives birth in a secluded northern- or eastern-facing room, and the house is completely shuttered, with the doors barred right through labour and for a good part of the following lying-in time.

In eastern Mediterranean countries women often used the communal bathhouse, where they were accustomed to gather together to relax, exchange news and reinforce female bonds.

An Ojibway baby was born in the birth hut constructed by the father a week or so before the due date, decided on a time scale of 'moons' since her last menstrual period. Choosing a place near running water, he dug a depression in the ground and built a curved hut of white cedar over it. This hut was called the 'tree of life'. He fixed a clutching pole above the dip in the ground, and when labour started the depression was filled with soft, fluffy fern fronds over which the mother could kneel or squat.

In rural areas in Japan the woman herself built the birth hut. It had to be dim inside, because the coming and going of the soul needed a dark place, and birth required the participation of spiritual powers. The *Kojiki*, the classic book of Japanese legend and history written in 712 AD, tells how the sea-god's daughter, her Augustness Luxuriant-Jewel Princess, built her birth hut at the sea's edge and thatched it with cormorant feathers.

In territory that women themselves control the mother has a sense of belonging, so that she can relax and trust her body to work, surrounded by familiar objects and sounds, and be with women who are close to her, rather than those employed by an institution. It is not only the things she sees – the branches of a tree outside her window swaying in the wind, a log fire burning in the grate, children coming in and out – but the sounds that she can hear – goats being driven to pasture, children coming home from school, neighbours chatting, birds in the garden. The birth is part of the rhythm of her life.

The traditional birth place presents a marked contrast to the modern hospital delivery room, which is usually busy, brightly lit, and often noisy. The woman is virtually on display, exposed on a bed or delivery table in the centre, surrounded by technical equipment, and, although female midwives offer immediate care and record progress, a male obstetrician is usually at the apex of the pyramid of authority and makes the ultimate diagnosis and decisions. When these midwives who have been trained in hospitals attend home births, they tend to take the hospital practices with them.

> *If a midwife uses the medicalised model of care at a home birth, such as restricted maternal nutritional intake, regular vaginal examinations, restricted maternal position, enforced pushing, amniotomy and so on, she will re-create the maternal and fetal distress of the hospital in the home where there is no back-up nearby.*[2]

Sheryl Feldman, a midwife who works with Amish women in Pennsylvania, who give birth in hospital or at home, writes about Pennsylvania Hospital in Philadelphia:

> *To the left, as one enters the unit, are cubbyholes, each one equipped with a bed and a fetal monitor. The laboring woman, we are told, will position herself on one of the beds in order to have a sample 'strip' taken on the fetal monitor. It establishes that she is indeed in labor and also provides a base for later comparisons. Her vagina is inspected with a speculum (a metal instrument) and her vital signs are measured and recorded. Those women who have had babies before and have no apparent complications are assigned to labor rooms to the front of the unit; the others are referred to the back of the unit to be nearer the delivery and operating rooms.*

> *To get to their rooms women pass by the nurses' station. It's a long, low, white module which, with its computer screen overhead, provokes thoughts of space launchings. Behind the desk is a bank of glass-faced shelves stacked with boxes of needles, syringes, exam gloves, and the like. A phone installation spreads across the center of the desk and its buttons buzz and flash.*

> *From behind the nurses' station one can see directly into four of these labor rooms. Each is about as wide as a subway car and about a third as long. The walls are green and illuminated by fluorescent light. Cramped up next to the bed is a stainless steel trolley and a confusion of equipment. We're told that the noncomplicated woman who labors in these rooms may have three to five attachments made to her. She will have a 'lock' put in her arm, which means she can be given fluids, drugs, and blood intravenously, having only to be punctured once. There's the datascope for the epidural, the belts for the fetal monitor, the Pitocin on a pump, and possibly oxygen. If she's uncomfortable and not on continuous monitoring, she can get up and walk around. At the moment, no one is taking advantage of this opportunity.*

Riding on a metal gurney, a woman near delivery breaks through swinging doors and into a corridor banked on either side by carts heaped with green sheets and stacked with stainless steel receptacles. Passing through another swinging door, she rides onto the delivery room floor, which is black and nubby, like a parking lot. To her left, nearly wall to wall, ceiling to floor, are metal drawers and cabinets, to her right, tables, warming lights, an isolette, instruments wrapped in packs. Blocking a window is a metal installation. It has tubes hanging from it, a bellows in a jar, buttons, switches, cords. A vast mirror and huge orange lights, like satellites, loom over the delivery table.[3]

With the introduction of modern hospitals women's birth places, space which belongs to them, which they themselves have created and where they control what happens, have often been despised or forgotten, even in isolated areas, and women are transported by car, boat or plane, sometimes for vast distances, to deliver in the city.

Among the Inuit of northern Canada it is believed that babies who are born far away from their homes cannot belong to their people in the same way as those born in the traditional birthplace. They have been dispossessed.

In Fiji, some women who travelled to deliver their first babies in hospital on the main island told me that they chose to give birth at home in the traditional way with other babies because the hospital experience was too stressful. They described feelings similar to those of women in Europe and North America who are haunted by the memory of traumatic births. Where traditional birth styles remain a possibility, they, unlike many women in exclusively technocratic birth systems, can plan for the next birth confident that it will be different. Some of the professional nurses based in village communities are working closely with traditional midwives to give women this option.

Western birth culture has had an insidious effect, sometimes positive, but often damaging, on what happens all over the world, wherever midwives in poverty-stricken developing countries are taught the most up-to-date styles of the management of birth by educators representing the advanced nations of the west. Old customs are destroyed and in birth cultures where women used to squat or kneel to give birth, they are no longer allowed to do so. In Guatemala today there are midwives who refuse to deliver a woman who is not lying down. Where women were accustomed to give birth on moss or ferns, or sun-baked sand, they now do so on plastic sheets. In India, because these cost 50 rupees each, *dais* re-use them, or, even cheaper, collect old agricultural fertiliser bags to deliver on instead.[4]

The violent management of birth that is characteristic of the medical–surgical model of a technocratic culture brings new dangers to traditional birth cultures. The introduction of uterine stimulants into a woman's bloodstream through a hypodermic syringe comes to be seen as a magic solution to a slow labour and tends to be employed indiscriminately, even routinely.

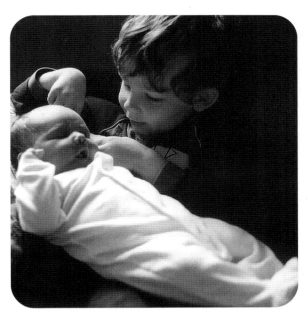

After the birth: a big brother welcomes the new baby and gently strokes his head

When all this is combined with a birth place that has changed radically from a domestic setting to a caricature of a modern hospital, a rusted iron delivery table, lithotomy stirrups, crumbling walls and chipped equipment, with flies buzzing around and bags of rubbish waiting to be emptied, it can be lethal.

Some courageous pioneering midwives in northern industrial countries are reaching out to help traditional and trained midwives in other cultures, opening up birth centres and changing care so that it takes on the best of the old and the new. Beatrice Carla is one such midwife. She started the Nepal Midwives' Initiative 'working with Nepali colleagues to replace outdated western-imported methods with an evidence-based, humane, holistic approach to labour and birth care'. In the Birth Centre in Kathmandu women can move around in labour and give birth in upright positions, and the episiotomy rate there is 15% compared with a national rate of 70–95%.[5]

Maternity hospitals were originally built in northern countries as places where very poor women could have their babies while simultaneously providing clinical material for the doctors and their students. The most dangerous place to give birth was in these hospitals, where death rates for babies and mothers were high. Even if a mother did not die during the birth, she was exposed to the risk of puerperal fever afterwards. Between the years 1860 and 1864, 9886 women were admitted to the Paris Maternité. Of these, 1226 mothers died, a mortality rate of 12.4%. It was a good deal safer to give birth at home, even if home was a slum, and to be attended by a midwife.[6]

Michel Odent believes that the best setting in which to give birth is similar to that in which to fall asleep. He writes about 'falling in labour' and compares it with 'falling to sleep'.[7]

In my own work I have suggested that the ideal environment for birth is like that for making love. They are both psycho-sexual activities in which the release of oxytocin and endorphins are stimulated. These are obstructed when there is embarrassment, lack of confidence, a feeling of having to put on a performance, fear or doubt.[8]

In a familiar domestic environment women use their surroundings for physical support and mobility. There is no specialised unfamiliar equipment to encounter. They are accustomed to using tables, chairs, window ledges, horizontal bars that can be gripped, a curtained four-poster bed, a large bag of rice or a futon, a milking stool, a wooden barrel, a hammock or rope slung from the rafters, a roller towel tied to a post, a rocking chair, a branch of a tree, or the central house pillar. They use immersion in warm water, hot mud or leaf packs, heated stones or a hot water bottle, to relieve pain during menstruation as well as in birth. There is a significant difference between handling pain in these ways and having medication for pain relief in the modern hospital.

Within the woman's own environment, she is in control. She makes decisions helped by other women who are all familiar with birth, just as they are with baking bread, cooking traditional dishes, grinding corn, doing their laundry by the river, weaving or plaiting, and curing the family's aches and pains. It is part of their cultural heritage.

Today, within a technocratic birth culture, some of us are exploring ways of changing the birth place so that it once again belongs to the mother, enabling her to move without constriction, to have privacy, and to focus her energies on birth-giving in a dimly lit, flexible and peaceful environment, one in which she can respond spontaneously to the power released in her body. The redesign of the birth place is not merely a matter of cosmetic changes to make it appear more homely, with a rocking chair, a patchwork quilt, pictures on the walls, and soft furnishings, a TV set and a jacuzzi. A birth place is the woman's own space in which she can trust her body and give birth with loving support in a way that she feels is right for her.[9]

References

1. Kitzinger S 2000 Rediscovering birth. London: Little Brown
2. Anderson T 2002 Out of the laboratory: back to the darkened room. MIDIRS Midwifery Digest 12(1):65–69
3. Armstrong P, Feldman S 1990 A wise birth. New York: Morrow, p 49
4. Kitzinger S 2000 Rediscovering birth. London: Little Brown
5. Nepal Midwives' Initiative, 5 Laverock Bank Terrace, Edinburgh EH5 3BJ
6. Lancet 1879;i:746–747
7. Odent M 2002 The farmer and the obstetrician. London: Free Association Books, pp 86–89
8. Kitzinger S 1983 Women's experience of sex. London: Dorling Kindersley
9. Kitzinger S 2002 Birth your way. London: Dorling Kindersley

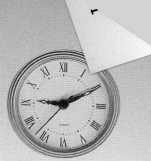

3
The clock, the bed and the chair

Many interventions accepted as normal in labour and birth are insidious and hallowed by time. They do not proclaim themselves with new technology, or entail major expenditure, but form part of the conventional environment of birth in northern industrial countries. Without them some caregivers would feel unsettled. They provide the basis of other interventions and are unrecorded because they are unseen.

The bed

Since the 1970s research has revealed that mobility enables the uterus to contract more efficiently and reduces perception of pain.[1–9] Yet in birth rooms around the world a bed is the central piece of furniture and is taken for granted. A bed is for getting into. It implies a certain kind of posture and a certain attitude of mind. Beds are for resting in, for easing aches and pains, and in a hospital for putting the body on display under professional gaze in order to examine, diagnose and manipulate it. Attendants gather round the bed and look down on it, lights are directed onto it, and equipment is lined up to connect with the body lying on it. The patient's body belongs to the bed, and the bed to the body. Bed-bound birth is perceived as normal, even inevitable, in the majority of hospitals everywhere. Any variation on this style of birth is seen as innovative and daring.

The clock

Another central item of equipment is the clock on the wall. It is often situated opposite the body on the bed. Birth records are based on the information it provides: the timing and length of contractions, assessment of uterine activity and cervical dilatation, the parameters of the first, second and third stages, and the Apgar score of the baby.

For some caregivers a birth without a clock would seem a shambles. They would feel out of control. The information produced by the clock is reinforced by the caregiver's watch and a print-out of an electronic fetal monitor which also records time. Labour and delivery are described in terms of the clock: membranes ruptured, intravenous catheter inserted, descent of the fetal head, medication given, infant and placenta delivered at specific times.

The active management of labour, as instituted in Dublin, which has now spread round the world, restricts labour and birth to time protocols dictated by the medical system.[10] Where active management is practised, any labour exceeding 12 hours is labelled 'failure to progress' and steps are taken to deliver instrumentally or by caesarean section. Indeed, a limit of 10 or even 8 hours is often imposed, and in Ireland a midwife attending a home birth is instructed to transfer her patient to hospital once this time limit is reached. Within a technocratic birth model, management cannot handle anything that is outside the designated time framework.

Even where active management is not practised, the key point and definitive marker is the time of the onset of the second stage, and, along with the length of the first stage, this has a profound effect on whether or not a woman has an instrumental delivery, a caesarean section or a spontaneous vaginal birth.

The atmosphere in many delivery rooms is like that of a wrestling match in which a highly charged audience enthusiastically shouts 'Come on! Come on! Go on! Push! You can do it!' Midwives often call out instructions to 'Push into your bottom', sometimes even 'Get angry with the baby!' The woman is cajoled, urged, commanded to push as hard and as long as she can – and then more. This is not only unphysiological and exhausting, but it may lead to torn cervical ligaments and vulval and perineal tissues, possible rectovaginal fistula, the risk to the mother of hypertension and stroke, and for the baby a reduction in the oxygen supply and also the risk of deep transverse arrest.[11] This method of conducting the second stage turns birth into a race against time, and can be counterproductive.

Clock-watched labour is so normal that it is unremarked.

The clock is an unevaluated technological intervention that has major impact on the conduct of birth.

Birth time at home and in hospital

In the narratives of hospital birth women frequently shape their accounts and rate the experience as easy or difficult with reference to the clock. When I analysed the language of birth stories narrated by women who delivered in hospital compared with those who had home births, it emerged that they made references to time in contrasting ways.

In hospital, birth time was recorded in relation to the clock and the partogram. Sometimes it is clear from the accounts that time dominated the decisions about labour. Everything that occurred happened at specific times, and some women even wrote their stories in the form of a time chart, with the exact time introducing each line or section. Home births were described in relation to natural phenomena, to night and day, dawn and dusk, full light, half-light and darkness, and also with reference to social relationships that impinged on the labour: children waking up, going to school, coming home, neighbours mowing the lawn or dropping in, and family mealtimes. One woman recorded that she found time to plant out beans in her garden, with the help of her midwife, before labour became too strong to do this any longer. Many home birth mothers told how they prepared meals in advance or baked a cake for the party afterwards.

When a woman was transferred from home to the hospital the decision was usually made in relation to time. One woman told how the midwife, who arrived at their home at 3 p.m., announced 'You must have this baby by 6 o'clock, because I'm going off duty then, and there's no one to take over from me'. Since she was still in labour at that time, the woman was transferred to hospital, labour was stimulated by a syntocinon intravenous drip, and she ended up with an emergency caesarean section on the grounds that labour was prolonged.

My mother described to me the long drawn out labour she experienced when she gave birth to me. There was a woodpecker in the tree outside her bedroom window, and the bird kept tapping throughout the labour: 'I thought if that little bird can keep working away at the hard wood, I can keep going, too'.

There are exceptions to this. A woman who sent me a record of a home birth in which times were carefully recorded, seemed to be aware that this account was unusual for a home birth. She explained that during labour they had no sense of time. It did not matter. They were caught up in the moment. But afterwards, as they organised the experience in a way that was presentable to other people, they used the times on their video camera with which her partner had filmed the birth to work out in retrospect exactly when everything occurred.

In traditional birth cultures time is perceived in a similar way to that in most of the home births I studied. There are the sounds of women going to market or down to the river to do laundry, of men returning from the fields, or the call of the *muezzin*, the aroma of a meal being cooked, and changes in the sky as time passes. Understanding of this by professional health educators is reflected in the pictorial report cards given to *paradeiras* (literally, the women who catch babies) in north-west Brazil. The hour of birth is recorded on a chart that shows pictures of sunrise, high sun, sunset and night.

Activity and stillness

In a technocratic culture care is segmented, with different professionals responsible for various tasks, both in pregnancy and in labour. The emphasis is on what birth professionals *do*, not on who they are as people and the atmosphere in the birth room. It is all about being busy. When we describe births in other cultures we often dissect them in the same way. What is everyone doing? In this way we miss the rhythms of birth. Perhaps this is because we have not been educated to observe pauses in action and spaces. In traditional cultures midwives still define birth in social terms rather than as medical processes.

In a technocratic culture time is measured. There are clear beginnings and endings and tasks that are performed, and these can all be recorded on a partogram and record chart. Midwifery is explained in terms of activity and intervention, not in terms of inaction or actions that seem to us, as outsiders, irrelevant to the progress of the birth. Yet the positive effect of a midwife's presence may be as much in stillness as in action.

The chair

When caregivers get women down off the bed other equipment tends to be offered. Rather than open space, a stool or chair is provided. Studies have been published from the 1980s, comparing use of a chair or stool with bed birth. None have been carried out comparing chair or stool with completely free movement. Whenever a chair or stool is used, or any other apparatus, it conveys the implicit message 'You sit here, place your feet there and grasp this'. The more elaborate the equipment, and the fewer the options available to the woman, the more it restricts movement.

Birth stools and chairs have a long history.[12] The medieval birth stool was a horseshoe- or boomerang-shaped slab of wood on legs, without a back and without arms. A woman could sit on it and move her pelvis freely. One of the god-sibs (women birth companions) sat behind her, cradling her against her

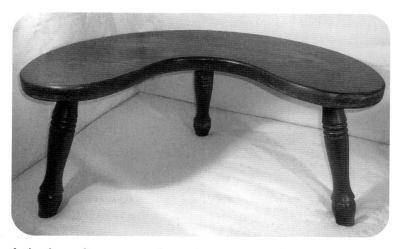

A simple, craftsperson-made, contemporary wooden birth stool

body and moving with her. It was a familiar, comfortable posture, since women were accustomed to sitting crouched on a low stool when milking a cow or goat and spinning or weaving.

The birth stool is a development of the birth bricks that were used in Egypt, Persia and India, and of lap-sitting, common throughout Africa, Europe and South America. A German father devised the birth stool with a back to it after his wife told other pregnant women in her neighbourhood how easy it had been giving birth sitting between her husband's thighs. As a result, women asked him to attend them when they were in labour and he became very popular in the town, to such a degree that he built a birth stool to take his place.

One version of the birth stool was elongated so that a woman could sit on it behind the mother, supporting her with her body. Only later were solid backs added to birth stools, and subsequently footplates and hand grips.

A variation, combining lap-sitting and a stool, was developed in the North American colonies in the 18th century. The woman sat between her husband's thighs on a stool turned on its side. She could move her pelvis and her women helpers sat in front of her so that she could reach and clasp their hands. This permitted more movement, with flexible support, than did a complicated birth stool. Stools became increasingly complicated, with padding, skirting and footrests, and by the 19th century had evolved into chairs that resembled domestic chairs in middle-class homes, often with extra decorative carving.

Some birth chairs were very elaborate. A cushioned chair was designed by a French *accoucheur* in the 18th century, for example, that masqueraded as an easy chair in a lady's boudoir, with a removable cut-out section beneath the vulva and a sliding tray that could be slotted back to allow the obstetrician closer access. It was called 'the bed of misery'. Many chairs had ratchets in the backrest so that the woman could be put into a reclining position.

From there it was only a matter of angle to tip her backward with her legs raised and pinioned. The activity of the labouring woman was now replaced by the activity of the *accoucheur*, and from then on birth chairs and tables were designed to facilitate obstetric manoeuvres without hindrance from the patients.

Squatting and kneeling positions have remained some of the most common postures in traditional cultures throughout the world. When I was doing research in a large Jamaican hospital in the 1960s, there was a running battle between labouring women and midwives. The women wanted to get up and crouch down, knees bent, and rock their pelvis forward and back, and the midwives were determined to get them on the bed or delivery table where they were expected to lie still and be good patients.

Birth chairs today have been re-invented. They range from simple low chairs with a cut-out horseshoe shape in the seat, to highly elaborate constructions that can be turned instantly into a delivery table complete with lithotomy stirrups or for caesarean section.

The simplest of contemporary birth chairs, as distinct from stools, used by some midwives in English birth centres, are made of metal with a cut-out seat, arms and a ridged back. The height of the seat cannot be adjusted, the arms are restricting and the solid back prevents pelvic mobility. Their only advantage seems to be that they enable a woman to be in an upright position. The elegant Roma chair, Swiss designed, and clearly 'woman-centred' with its circular loops and springy, cushioned seat, suggests activity because it resembles a piece of athletic equipment. But it has footrests that indicate where a woman should place her feet. She can press against or pull on the metal bars that soar above her, but cannot kneel, squat or get on all fours.

In theory, a pool allows a woman, supported by water, to move unencumbered. Or so it might be thought. Although published research often refers to mobility as an advantage of being in a pool, some birth pools are elaborate constructions with seats, handgrips and footrests, and movement in them is restricted.[13] Any pool designed as a tub for the frail and elderly is, by its nature, confining. Equally, a pool embellished with a built-in moulded plastic stool, a ramp, foot supports, shower and handles can be equally restrictive.

When a woman uses a birth stool or chair, or is in a pool, it cannot be assumed that she moves freely. Comparative research is needed in which video is used to record the range of positions and movements women actually adopt when labouring and giving birth on birth stools, chairs or in a pool. Video can also be used to record the interaction between the midwife and mother, to reveal whether the caregiver suggests specific positions and movements or enables the mother to take the lead.

Medical equipment firms that manufacture modern birth chairs emphasise in their promotional material that electronic controls are under the command of the obstetrician. At the flick of a switch or pressure on a button he can either enable the woman to squat grasping a birth bar, with space on her perineum so that it can be guarded, and rotation of the baby's head manually assisted, or he can tip the woman into the Trendeleberg position, or have her flat on her back for an instrumental delivery or caesarean section. Contemporary birth chairs are, in the final resort, under the control of the obstetrician.

References

1. Liu YC 1974 Effects of an upright position during labor. American Journal of Nursing 74(12):2202–2205

2. Flynn A, Kelly J, Hollins G, Lynch PF 1978 Ambulation in labour. BMJ 2:591–593

3. Caldeyro-Barcia R 1979 The influence of maternal position on time of spontaneous rupture of the membranes, progress of labor and fetal head compression. Birth 6:10–18

4. de Jong PR, Johanson RB, Baxen P, et al 1997 Randomised trial comparing upright and supine positions for the second stage of labour. British Journal of Obstetrics and Gynaecology 104(5):567–571

5. Diaz AG, Schwartz R, Fescina R, et al 1980 Vertical position during the first stage of the course of labor and neonatal outcome. European Journal of Obstetrics, Gynecology and Reproductive Biology 11(1):1–7

6. Chamberlain G, Stewart M 1987 Walking through labour. BMJ 295(6602):802

7. Roberts J 1989 Maternal position during the first stage of labour. In: Chalmers I, Enkin M, Keirse MJNC (eds) Effective care in pregnancy and childbirth, vol 2. Oxford: Oxford University Press, pp 883–892

8. Sleep J, Roberts J, Chalmers I 1989 Care during the second stage of labour. In: Chalmers I, Enkin M, Kierse MJNC (eds) Effective care in pregnancy and childbirth, vol 2. Oxford: Oxford University Press, pp 1130–1134

9. Gupta, J, Nikodem C 2000 Maternal posture in labour [review]. European Journal of Obstetrics, Gynecology and Reproductive Biology 92(2):273–277

10. Thornton JG 1997 Active management of labour [review]. Current Opinion in Obstetrics and Gynecology 9(6):366–369

11. Sleep J, Roberts J, Chalmers I 1989 Care during the second stage of labour. In: Chalmers I, Enkin M, Kierse MJNC (eds) Effective care in pregnancy and childbirth, vol 2. Oxford: Oxford University Press, pp 1130–1134

12. Engelmann G 1882 Labor among primitive peoples. St. Louis: Chambers. E-book available at: http://www.etext.lib.virginia.edu/toc/modeng/public/EngLabo.html (accessed 4 November 2004)

13. Burns E, Kitzinger S 2001 Midwifery guidelines for use of water in labour. Oxford: School of Health and Social Care, Oxford Brookes University

4

Images of birth and breastfeeding

Visual images of birth and breastfeeding shape the way we think about these experiences and express key values of our culture.

Every society has its birth culture, just as it has a culture of kinship relations, food and eating, dealing with illness, all the important activities of daily life, transitions between different stages of life, and the rites surrounding death. In clay, drawings and paintings, in sacred places, medical textbooks, today in the literature of health promotion and in the media, the ways in which birth and breastfeeding are represented give us clues to their meanings in each culture.

Birth

Since Palaeolithic times, human birth has never been considered merely a biological act. In societies all over the world it has symbolised the coming into being of every living thing. The first birth is the origin of all life. God gives birth, mountains and seas are formed, and people, animals and plants are created. Each birth links the present with the past and future of humanity. It has spiritual significance. Carved in rock in caves that are the womb of Mother Earth, geometric signs represent a woman's body heavy with pregnancy and the momentous process of birth. In the caves of south-west France archaeologists have discovered rock carvings of women, and it has been suggested that women gave birth in niches in these caves, with fire burning at the entrance to keep bears and other predators away.

Women have constructed clay images of birth in cultures across the world. Universally, these show the mother giving birth in an upright position. She is

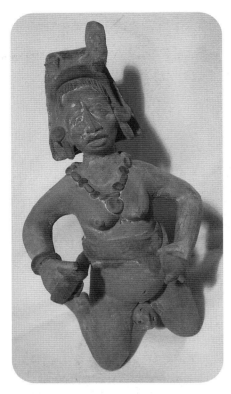

A birth sculpture of a Mexican mother kneeling, rocking and using her *rebozo* to press on the fundus

often attended by at least one other woman, and there may be two, one supporting her from behind and the other kneeling in front. In Peru and Mexico, the Canadian Arctic, throughout Africa, and on the islands of the Pacific these birth sculptures recur. Indian tribal sculptures in Bihar, for example, show the mother kneeling on the ground, other women physically supporting her, and the *dai* assisting at the birth and pressing her feet against her inner thighs.

In the Christian tradition the births of St. John and of Mary, the mother of Jesus, were a popular Renaissance image in religious paintings. In Medieval Europe, too, a woman called on female friends when she went into labour. They came to help, took over the house, and often stayed for weeks after the birth. There was a party atmosphere, and a great deal of food and alcohol was consumed. These women were known as 'god-sibs', literally 'sisters in God'. In male language the term 'god-sib' became changed to 'gossip'. In the Renaissance paintings of the births of St. John and Mary the moments after birth were shown, never the birth itself, and there were always women helpers attending the mother and bathing or swaddling the baby. There is a bustle of female activity. Men are absent.

Images of the birth of Jesus, the kind that often appear on Christmas cards today, were a complete contrast. There were no helping women, only the animals quietly watching, and Joseph, who was quite obviously out of place, either detached from the scene and praying, or frightened and embarrassed. It was not so much poverty as the absence of helping women that made this a birth distinct from all others. The focus is on Mary's social isolation. The absence of woman-to-woman love and care is perceived as a terrible deprivation.

German woodcuts of the 16th century, including some by Durer, show a woman on a birth stool assisted by a midwife, and other women physically supporting the mother and preparing a celebratory feast to follow the birth. Occasionally, a man is present in the background or at the door, his back turned, examining the heavens to predict the baby's future from the position of the stars.

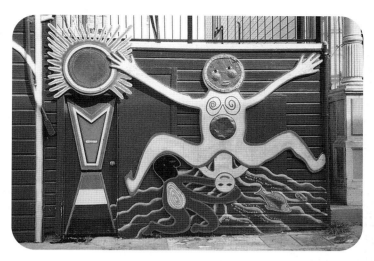

Brilliantly coloured birth art on a wall in San Francisco's Mission District

After this, birth was rarely the subject of European art until a genre of birth paintings flourished in The Netherlands depicting the time immediately following birth. The Dutch scenes show a comfortable and prosperous domestic setting, and focus on the social nature of birth, with visiting family, friends and neighbours. In place of the bustling groups of busy women typical of paintings of the Italian Renaissance. There are grandparents and other relatives quietly admiring the baby, drinking coffee and eating cakes.

Medical representations of birth

In 16th century France, Italy and Germany, drawings of women in childbirth were first employed for medical studies. They took the form of classical nudes in erotic poses or Eve holding an apple, the woman's insides ripped open and the fetus shaped like that of a miniature adult.

In the 18th century anatomical models made in wax (and later terracotta) were first used in medical studies in Italy. The woman was constructed so that her body parts could be lifted out in layers and she was depicted as a courtesan, or fallen woman, pearls at her throat and her hair often unbound. In the Bologna Wax Museum and in museums in Florence and Vienna, glass cases reveal these wax figures of pregnant women, reclining and abandoned, heads thrown back, in sadomasochistic display. Models like these were also commissioned for private collections.

They figure the erotic plots of romance, types of the seductress and adulteress that people late 18th and 19th century novels, their sexual allure and power

25

managed by making them objects to be exposed and manipulated. Their bodies are crafted to open, layer after layer, organ after organ, until a fetus is revealed.[1]

Professor Karen Newman points out that in these wax figures and drawings anatomical violence is eroticised 'by surrounding the open body with drapery and leaving intact ... the breasts and pubic hair'. In William Hunter's drawings, in contrast, the fetus 'is wedged unbearably not into a woman's body – Eve, Venus, odalisque – but, spectacularly, into meat'.[2] His illustrations look like drawings in Mrs Beeton's cookery book, showing how to carve a joint.

By the beginning of the 19th century, birth scenes had disappeared almost entirely from art and were found only in the pages of medical texts, with detailed drawings of obstetric manoeuvres. Many of these are American. The woman has become a patient who is placed in various positions for easy access by the obstetrician. She is usually headless, may be limbless, and the detached arm of the doctor manipulates the baby's head. He wears a suit with immaculately white, starched cuffs and discreet cufflinks. In these textbooks a nurse appears who is splaying the patient's legs and holding her in position so that the physician can perform his sleight of hand. The whole emphasis is on pathology. The obstetrician is the star of the show, and the mother is completely passive. The living, breathing woman is spectacularly absent. Instead, there is a lump of body that might just as well be that of a corpse.

Today, at conferences of midwives and obstetricians where firms that manufacture medical equipment display their goods, the female body during parturition may be represented as a pink plastic dummy, bits of which can be unscrewed or lifted off to reveal internal organs. Inside one model there is a fetus – permanently extended with outstretched legs and a head that cannot be flexed onto the chest – which is propelled mechanically down through the cervix and a stockinette pelvic floor that looks more like a car windscreen cloth than human tissue. There is a rigid plastic vulva into which an examining and manipulating hand can be

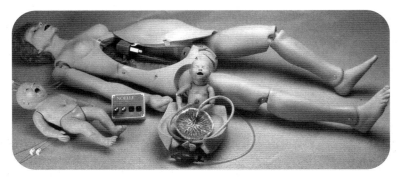

The NOELLE Simulator with an 'automatic birthing system'
(Reproduced with permission of Gaumard Scientific)

introduced. But the mother is spectacularly missing both clitoris and anus, or a woman at the other end who stiffens with pain, withdraws from physical contact, or screams when hurt. She is without heart, blood vessels or blood. She has no lungs, no stomach and no diaphragm.[3] She is the epitome of reproductive female minus all the parts that do not matter. She lies supine, unable to sit up or roll over, or to squat, kneel or stand. She is simply an object on which the obstetrician acts, and on which a catheter can be passed, a fetal head rotated, or a fetus extracted by forceps, ventouse or caesarean section. At one hospital a microphone has been added connecting with another room, where someone can introduce the sounds that are lacking, and after midwives and others (including me) contacted the manufacturer to complain about the lack of authenticity of a fetus that could not bend its head it is being redesigned with a more flexible head.

In the 1920s the first books about birth written for mothers came on the market. Grantly Dick-Read's *Revelation of Childbirth* was published, the second edition of which was entitled *Childbirth Without Fear*. This included fuzzy photographs of women doing antenatal exercises and in labour, the first time such photographs had appeared. A black rectangle masked each woman's face. This had the effect of turning her into a body without a brain or personality.

Today most images of birth directed at the public are either for a specific audience – pregnant women – or are confronted on the TV screen. The jackets of 'how to' books for expectant mothers, including my own, avoid representing birth. Instead there is a blonde mother with a baby in her arms, a radiant pregnant woman walking by the sea, or a cuddly baby. Publishers steer clear of showing birth pictures on the cover, believing that it might offend potential readers.

But birth has found a place in the marketing of some products, precisely because of its ability to shock. There is the Benneton advertisement that showed a naked, screaming newborn, cord still uncut, and an Italian shoe advertisement revealing the splayed legs of a woman who is wearing stylish high-heeled sandals, with her feet in lithotomy stirrups. The baby is suspended upside-down, and a delivery team, all masked, are admiring either the baby, the shoes – or perhaps both.

Embroidered representations of birth in Judy Chicago's dinner table portrayal of childbirth shock in a different way. Here the vagina is represented as a ripped fissure, an agonised split. It portrays the suffering of birth – the woman is an iconic figure, legs and arms splayed, analogous with that of Christ on the cross. The focus is on the drama and pain of birth.

On TV, programmes about reproductive medicine are popular. In a biomedical documentary, a member of the House of Lords in a multi-coloured Velcro suit is repeatedly throwing himself against a Velcro-lined wall. This is 'Superhuman: the work of the baby-builders', and Lord Winston is a fertilised ovum attempting to implant in the uterine wall. Then the camera closes in on a vigorous crop of fungi, and Lord Winston raises the hope that we shall 'grow human eggs as easily as we now harvest mushrooms'. In these science documentaries on British TV it is always the dominant male who is doing the innovative construction and harvesting work and who turns barrenness to fertility and female failure to fulfilment: the reproductive scientist as Prospero.

Another series, *The Body Story*, shows the embryo as a scheming alien, which first takes endocrine control over the mother's whole physiological system and then ruthlessly exploits her body in its own interest. She is perceived as victim, passively suffering the fetal conquest.

In situation comedies (sit-coms) birth is treated humorously, with strong emphasis on the incompetent father who panics as soon as the woman has her first contraction, and birth is treated with high drama in hospital serials that explore the love–hate relationships of doctors, nurses and other personnel and the emotional lives of patients who are snatched from disaster.

TV comedy and drama programmes, many of which are exported all over the world from the USA, represent pregnancy and birth as leading to social embarrassment, highly stressed personal relationships, and often chaos. The father is picked out to be a figure of fun. He tends to say and do all the wrong things. He panics and drives off without the woman, takes the wrong one to hospital, then keels over, and the nurses (they are usually nurses, not midwives) have to tend him instead of the woman in labour.

The start of labour is signalled by sudden, agonising pain around the navel. The woman clutches her bump with a look of shocked horror on her face and is immediately immobilised, remaining in that state more or less until the baby is born. With each pain she clutches her abdomen again. On TV women rarely have backache labour. The pain is always at the top of their tummies – an unlikely site in most labours. Childbirth entails a desperate rush to get her to hospital. Everything else is irrelevant. She is like a parcel to be transported, pushed, pulled and dumped on a delivery table in front of a highly efficient, gowned (and often masked) medical team. The senior obstetrician cracks out staccato commands and a junior member, almost invariably a woman, makes soothing noises.

In a film called *Nine Months* the obstetrician is the comic star. Having recently arrived from Eastern Europe, he is expert in the birth of baboons rather than human birth, and is having difficulty with the English language ('Now I examine your Volvo'). The father is engaged in frenetic videoing of two births, his wife's and another's, and there is a fist-fight between the two fathers as the babies are delivered from under the mothers' heavily draped bodies.

In virtually all sit-coms birth is presented as an emergency from which women and babies can only be rescued by doctors. Analysis reveals that 26% of the mothers never make it to the hospital in time for the birth.[4] Babies are usually delivered by doctors, not midwives, although in reality in Britain a midwife is the senior person in the room at 68% of births.[5] Any hospital drama in which the mother expresses the hope that she will have a natural birth is a coded warning to the viewer that labour will be long and difficult, and that she or the baby may die. In an episode of *ER*, a woman who is already eclamptic says that she wants a natural birth. But she has to ask for an epidural, because the pain is too severe. Against a background of bleeping machines, and people running everywhere, there is shoulder dystocia, an emergency caesarean, massive haemorrhage, followed by stabilisation – but then she fits, and dies. Her partner is left sitting in a rocking chair, the baby in his arms, grieving over his wife.

Home births either occur in historical dramas, or take place by accident. One writer comments that 'TV heroines only ever give birth in lifts, taxis, beside remote lakes or in planes, three miles up above the Earth'.[6]

TV has produced a powerful mythology of birth. The drama of this myth is in the medical emergency, the speeding ambulance, the urgent bleep, and the struggles of a team of doctors and nurses to combat death. There are heart monitors on which the trace flattens out, caesarean deliveries, haemorrhages, resuscitation of the baby. It is a drama that feeds the fears inherent in the dominant medical model of birth and conditions pregnant women to submit to its ritual.

Breastfeeding

The image of the nurturing mother with a baby at her breast is central to Christianity. In art galleries around the world, and especially in Italy, this is a powerful symbol of maternal love. Yet there was a much earlier pagan goddess who suckled the infant Horus, and goddesses are similarly represented in African and Pacific island carvings breastfeeding their babies. The breastfeeding goddess is a universal image. The lactating breast conveys the message of fertility and life-giving sustenance. It represents pure love – a woman giving herself to her child, the Great Mother nurturing her people.

Today, this image coexists with, and has been superseded by, other representations of the breast as sexually arousing. A press item in 2004 reported how a woman who was breastfeeding her baby in a London art gallery rich with images of the Virgin Mary breastfeeding the Christ child was asked to leave. The implicit message is that breasts are for the delectation of men rather than the feeding of babies, and exposed breasts symbolise a woman's sexual availability. When a woman breastfeeds openly in northern industrial culture she is often perceived as an exhibitionist, even as challenging men by offering a baby a part of her body that rightly belongs to them.

In the media breastfeeding is usually either invisible or presented negatively.[7] It is portrayed as a socially marginal activity, unlike bottle-feeding which is integrated into everyday scenes. It is rarely shown on TV, whereas bottle feeding is common. An analysis of programmes on British TV over a period of one month revealed a single scene of a baby being put to the breast. In contrast, 170 scenes showed babies' bottles, formula preparation or bottle-feeding.[4]

Babies' feeding bottles have become a routine and iconic way of visually representing babyhood, and are also used to symbolise positive male involvement in parenthood. For example, an advertisement for whisky shows a man in a dressing gown preparing formula. The strap line is 'What have you been doing while Bells whisky has been maturing?' Breastfeeding, by contrast, is portrayed as a slightly abnormal activity and is sometimes used to characterise particular types of women, for example 'hippies' or middle-class 'Earth mothers'.[4]

Bottle-feeding is usually represented as problem-free, whereas breastfeeding is fraught with difficulties. In both press and TV during that month of analysis there was only one reference to potential difficulties associated with bottle-feeding (the 'hassle' of sterilising bottles), but 42 references to difficulties attributed to nursing (sore nipples, 'saggy' breasts and sleepless nights). The entire month's sample had only one, oblique, TV reference to any potential disadvantages of formula feeding and a single newspaper feature that questioned the safety of genetically modified ingredients in a particular brand. The health benefits of human milk were never mentioned.[4]

In comedy programmes the humour exploits and reinforces ideas about the shame of leaking breasts, the 'disgusting' nature of breast milk and male double standards about 'tits' and 'boobs'. Most TV programmes that include anything about birth or breastfeeding display women's bodies as malfunctioning, polluting and dangerous. Women are by nature incontinent. Substances that ooze from our bodies are uncontrolled and polluting. Only under medical direction can we be rescued from disaster. Breastmilk is like menstrual blood, faeces, urine, phlegm.

Yet the media may be beginning to challenge this, at least with reference to breastfeeding. A British soap opera, *Brookside*, a drama series set in a Liverpool community, which was screened at peak time and attracted large audiences, ran a storyline about breastfeeding. One episode portrayed a businesswoman challenging objections to her breastfeeding in public. Her colleagues stood up for her right to do so, and the complainant, rather than she, was asked to leave the bar.

In the sit-com *Roseanne*, a US-made programme, the heroine was breastfeeding as she took her marriage vows. At the words 'You may kiss the bride', she declared 'Just let me change sides' and moved the baby to her other breast.

In *Friends* two men displayed embarrassment about breastfeeding. The baby's father, Ross, who had donated his sperm to the lesbian mother, claimed that it was 'the most beautiful, natural thing in the world'. One of the others commented 'Yes, but there's a baby sucking at it'. Another asked 'If the baby blows into one, does the other one get larger?' At this point the father was disgusted and got up in horror. The lesbian mother came in and asked Phoebe, 'How did it go?', she replied, 'I tasted your milk!' Rachael exclaimed 'That is juice squeezed from a person!' Ross blurted out 'Gross!' The mother said, 'My breastmilk is gross?' Ross steeled himself to taste it, swigged some down from the bottle, stuffed his mouth with cookies, and said, 'Not bad! It's like cantaloupe juice!' The story unfolded around the issue of purity and pollution, the goodness of breastmilk contrasted with disgust at an adult tasting it. Maybe TV images of breastfeeding have started to be subversive!

References

1. Newman K 1996 Fetal positions. Palo Alto, CA: Stanford University Press, pp 86–88

2. Newman K 1996 Fetal positions. Palo Alto, CA: Stanford University Press, pp 100–101

3. Noelle maternal and neonatal birthing simulator. Gaumard Scientific sales catalog: Miami, FL: Gaumard, 2004, p 44. Available at: http://www.gaumard.com

4. Clement S 1997 Childbirth on television. British Journal of Midwifery 5(1):37–42

5. Royal College of Midwives 2000 Evidence to the review body for nursing staff, midwives, health visitors and professions allied to medicine for 2001. London: Royal College of Midwives, p 21

6. Cobb J 1995 Birth on the box. New Generation 3–4

7. Henderson L, Kitzinger J, Green J 2000 Representing infant feeding: content analysis of British media portrayals of bottle feeding and breastfeeding. BMJ 321(7270):1196–1198

5

Breastfeeding: public health, birth and shame

Breastfeeding was already considered a public health issue in the USA in the mid-19th century. Normal practice was to breastfeed through to the end of the baby's second summer, because of the risk of diarrhoea in hot weather. Yet women who worked outside the home often could not do this. In Baltimore, the mortality rate was 59% higher than average for babies whose mothers worked outside the home and 5% lower than average for those who took in laundry or cooked meals for unmarried men. The working class stay-at-home mothers breastfed.[1]

In 1897, 18% of babies in Chicago died before their first birthday. The Chicago Department of Health estimated that 15 of those fed on cows' milk died for every one breastfed.[2]

In the 20th century, in a cogent analysis of infant feeding practices and public health campaigns in the USA, Jacqueline Wolf[2] states: 'The shift from breasts to bottle essentially redefined "normal" infant health. As early as the 1930s paediatricians deemed streams of respiratory, ear, and gastrointestinal infections inevitable childhood events'. Today in the USA 'Whether a physician or a physician's wife has breastfed is the best predictor of a doctor's ability and willingness to give accurate advice and appropriate support to lactating mothers'.[3] It is not so different in the UK. In spite of policies to promote breastfeeding, for many women access to sensible breastfeeding advice and emotional support for exclusive and extended breastfeeding is difficult to come by. But now this is rapidly being recognised as a public health issue.

For the sake of children's health – and for many in the developing world their very survival – the World Health Organisation (WHO) advises that babies should be exclusively breastfed for 6 months. Yet in the UK only 69% of babies born in 2000 were ever breastfed. By the time they were 4 months old, just 28% were still given any breast milk, and by 6 months only a meagre 21% were getting any breastmilk.[4]

In the USA the first national survey of women's childbearing experiences revealed that, although two-thirds of mothers intended to breastfeed exclusively, already by the end of the first week after birth only three in five were exclusively breastfeeding.[5] In this survey, 80% of the mothers said that they were given free formula samples, and 47% of the babies were provided with water or formula to supplement breastmilk.

Clearly, women need more support for breastfeeding. On the other hand, research into one-to-one support for breastfeeding mothers by trained volunteers revealed that it did not make it more likely that they continued breastfeeding after 6 weeks. In fact, even if mothers did breastfeed, they were likely to switch to the bottle at the same time as mothers given no extra support. While women said they valued the support of a counsellor, the availability of help did not increase breastfeeding rates.[6] Perhaps support has to be given in the first days after birth and continue one-to-one over the coming weeks, and maybe it should not be left to the women to seek help.

Becoming a mother turns life upside down. A woman may find it impossible to fit everything into the 24 hours, give time to breastfeed, and have any time for herself. Even good advice adds another burden. She often receives conflicting advice from friends, family and professionals who are trying to help. New mothers are counselled without recognition of the social context in which they are struggling to survive. Breastfeeding is never only a matter of technique – filling a baby up with milk just as the tank of a car is filled with petrol. Although it is vital that the baby has a good latch on the breast, even this is affected by how a woman feels about breastfeeding and how she thinks about her body. The way she handles the baby and whether or not she persists through difficulties depend on this perception.

Many women choose not to breastfeed because they live in a culture in which bottle-feeding is the norm. When I was doing research among Asian women in Bradford, I learned that these mothers bottle-fed, although some had previously breastfed babies successfully for 2 years or longer before arriving in the UK. I asked them why this was the case and invariably received the answer: 'We wish to do as *your* women do'. The environment which they saw as modern and progressive, representing all that an urban, industrialised society had to offer, was that of a northern working class they encountered in their limited excursions outside the home on their clinic visits. Many were virtually living in purdah – with the TV set. One of the first steps they made towards acculturation was the decision to bottle-feed.

Yet, even a woman who is determined to breastfeed often gives up in despair. Successful breastfeeding depends on confidence and a sense of self-worth.

The culture of childbirth has profound effects on how a woman feels about her body during the weeks and months after the baby is born. When birth is medicalised and she learns that it is dangerous for her to trust her body functions and that she must be continually screened to check for the presence of pathology, the whole childbirth experience tends to alienate her from her body. She can no longer rely on it to work naturally. This starts in pregnancy with screening procedures that may reveal a low-lying placenta and raise concerns about intra-uterine growth retardation, hypertension, gestational diabetes, malpresentation of the fetus and, finally, prolonged pregnancy that leads to induction of labour.

The labour itself further reduces her self-confidence. A long, tiring labour, with interventions to trigger the uterus into greater activity, leaves her feeling mauled and abused. A prolonged second stage in which she is urged to push harder and longer in a desperate attempt to get the baby out is not only exhausting, but destroys all her trust in her body. If she has epidural anaesthesia she may have no spontaneous impulse to push. So she is commanded to do so and surrounded by a cheer-leading team who urge her on in a race against time. It seems to her that her body just does not work as it should.

This can have a major impact on breastfeeding. To say that a managed labour with obstetric intervention lowers self-esteem is an understatement. If a mother has an instrumental delivery, the risk of which is greater with an epidural or a caesarean section, she may feel a failure as a woman. Other women can do it, why can't she?

Some new mothers, with the right kind of one-to-one support – consistent and sensitive to how they are feeling – triumph over all obstacles. But many do not.

Starting to breastfeed

Breastfeeding is sometimes discussed in isolation, and when this happens we trivialise or ignore the difficulties a new mother may be up against. Becoming a mother, the relationship with the baby, and breastfeeding are part of a continuum. The experience of birth has consequences not only for maternal and newborns' physical health, but for a woman's perceptions of herself as a human being and a mother, the baby's inborn skills at adapting to life, and the interaction between the mother and baby.[7] Anything that restricts postpartum contact between them makes breastfeeding more difficult.[7] This includes caesarean delivery, absence of skin-to-skin contact between mother and baby, removal of the baby to the nursery and not initiating breastfeeding in the first half hour or so after birth.

To these must be added all the interventions that pathologise labour, stress out the mother, and make an instrumental or caesarean delivery more likely. Mary Kroeger's book *Impact of Birthing Practices on Breastfeeding* is rich with information about these.[8]

Drugs for pain relief may affect both mother and baby. It is well known that, because they affect the central nervous system, opioids such as pethidine and meperidine, for example, can reduce a baby's alertness at and after birth.

Women are often told that an epidural has no effect on the baby. There is mounting evidence that this is not true. An American prospective, blinded, controlled study followed 129 mother and baby couples for 6 weeks after birth. Babies of mothers who had not had an epidural, rooted, latched on and sucked significantly better than the babies of epidural mothers. Both sets of mothers breastfed successfully, but the epidural mothers weaned their babies earlier.[9]

A Swedish paediatrician, Dr Lennart Righard, undertook research into breastfeeding behaviour immediately following birth, recording it on video. Most babies who have not been drugged creep to the breast, latch on and suck, but those who are drugged are unable to do this.[10] This study was followed by further research on the ways in which babies coordinate hand movements, moving their hands in the pauses in between suckling, and so stimulate the ejection of oxytocin in the mother.[11] Babies in the epidural group make hand-to-mouth movements, but are significantly less likely to touch the nipple, lick it, and latch on and suck. They are also more likely to have a raised temperature.

Another study[12] observed mothers and babies in two active breastfeeding sessions in the first 24 hours after birth. Breastfeeding went well in the first day after birth for 70% of the mother–baby couples who had an epidural, compared with 81% of the mother–baby couples who did not have an epidural. Babies of mothers who had an epidural were also more likely to be given a supplementary bottle of artificial baby milk while they were in hospital.

Some babies find it very difficult to latch on and are unable to coordinate sucking, swallowing and breathing. They may look as if they are sucking, but are not actually pressing on the milk glands. They can be very distressed, and the mother may say that she thinks her baby has a headache.

Linda Smith has a fascinating chapter in Mary Kroeger's book[13] called *Physics, Forces, and Mechanical Effects of Birth on Breastfeeding*, in which she points out that the baby's ability to suck, swallow and breathe while feeding is controlled by cranial nerves and around 60 muscles, acting on 22 bones in the baby's skull. She explains that mechanical forces during birth can disrupt the alignment of bony structures and affect nerve and muscle function. Instrumental birth and caesarean section produce additional mechanical forces on bony structures over and above the levels of force that occur in spontaneous vaginal birth.[13]

The hypoglossal nerve controls the baby's tongue movements that are needed for latching on and sucking. It lies in the space between segments of the occipital bone at the back of the baby's head. The nerve can become trapped, and this causes or contributes to disorganised or ineffective contraction of the tongue muscles. Other muscle fibres and nerves that lie between the segments of the occiput control muscles that are necessary for swallowing. If these are damaged, the suck–swallow–breathe reflexes are affected, and a gag response may be produced.

When a baby has a caput, which is to be expected after a ventouse extraction, venous return through the jugular vein and other blood vessels may also be obstructed. A study of babies who were delivered by vacuum extraction showed that breastfeeding was significantly more likely to be unsuccessful.[14]

Forceps delivery can also inhibit the baby's feeding reflexes. The trigeminal nerve may be damaged:

> *Motor fibers control the facial muscles, lips, cheeks, and jaw which are also directly involved in rooting, latching, and sucking responses. If the facial nerve is compromised, the infant may not be able to feel or respond to the breast in its mouth, nor use the tongue to grasp the nipple–areolar complex. Compromise to the motor fibers could result in using lip muscles to tightly grasp the nipple tip, instead of using tongue and intraoral muscles to grasp the nipple/areolar complex, thereby adversely affecting normal suck– swallow–breathe and comfortable, coordinated breastfeeding.*[13]

Caesarean delivery may not make it easier for the baby. It can also result in damage. The baby is usually lifted out by upward traction on the cranial base. This may damage the hypoglossal nerve running between the occipital plates. Babies who are born by caesarean are usually suctioned vigorously, too, and this

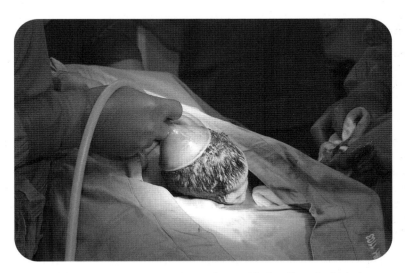

A vacuum extractor for caesareans. It moulds itself to the baby's head, does not form a chignon of traumatised tissue, but still requires powerful traction over the entire scalp cup
(Reproduced with permission of Mendox AB and Dickinson Healthcare Supplies)

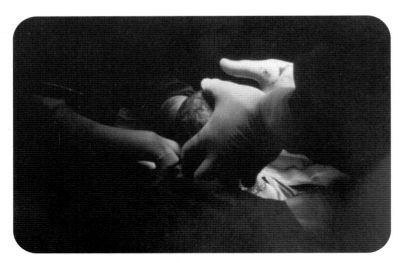

A caesarean: lifting the baby out by upward traction on the cranial base

can cause further damage. Any bruises and lacerations that produce oedema or haemorrhage may obstruct the baby's airway.

The author concludes: 'More research is urgently needed to confirm or rule out relationships between disorganised feeding and birth practices, events, and interventions'.

These difficulties can be surmounted, but it takes time. The mother's milk supply needs to be stimulated. Meanwhile, the baby needs to be hydrated and fed, either with its own or another mother's milk. The strong, sensitive and confident emotional support that a good midwife gives is vital. The chances are then that it is only a matter of time and self-confidence before breastfeeding becomes a satisfying and happy experience for both mother and baby.

Body image and the sense of self

In the days and weeks immediately following birth a woman's body is open, vulnerable and leaking. It feels soft and flabby. Her abdomen is loose and crumpled like a flat cream puff. Her perineum is sore and aching – and often mutilated by a deliberately inflicted surgical wound. It is difficult to sit with comfort. As her breasts become swollen and engorged, milk drips steadily out from her tender nipples. She may feel that everything about this experience is messy. The image that her body presents now is the polar opposite of the image of woman's bodies as they are presented in the media.

A common reason for women deciding to stop breastfeeding is that they feel 'used', 'drained' or 'exhausted'. Since many a breastfed newborn is a more or less continuous feeder, baby care can stretch out into what seems an endless ribbon of days and nights. Education in northern industrial cultures is geared towards task-oriented work and projects that can be performed one at a time, completed, and the results assessed. Being a mother, however, is not like this. She cannot do one thing at a time. The work is repetitive, and there is no certificate to show that she is doing well. It is hardly surprising that when a woman is trying to cope with this experience it is difficult to enjoy breastfeeding. She may feel sucked dry by an angry, screaming and incontinent tyrant. A woman who has no confidence in her body or her ability to be a mother may also feel that the baby does not really belong to her. Concerned people who are trying to help – the health visitor, her mother, her mother-in-law and other relatives – watch anxiously. When the baby cries the first question the mother is bound to get is 'Are you sure you have enough?' She looks at the milk and sees that it is watery and blue. She feels that it cannot really be good enough for the baby. It does not seem thick or rich enough.

For some women breastfeeding is sexually threatening, and they are frightened that it will destroy the mystery and romance in a relationship. If, as often happens, there is loss of libido after childbirth and, either because of a traumatic labour or a perineal wound, or simply because a woman feels connected to the baby by an invisible umbilical cord, she feels that to allow herself to enjoy breastfeeding is to take something away from her sexual partner. The man may resent the baby at the breast or be envious of the woman's power to give birth and to nurture a child.

The sexual threat of breastfeeding is to some extent a result of inadequate and lop-sided sex education. The emphasis is on intercourse as the one valid experience. Young people rarely learn that for a woman, anyway, sex is one part of passionate, tender relationships, and she is able to express love through her body in different ways. Breastfeeding is not merely 'parentcraft'.[15]

Judaeo-Christian culture sees the body as a container, the exits and entrances of which must be kept closed except on certain occasions when they are permitted to be opened, as Mary Douglas indicated in her book *Purity and Danger*.[16, 17] Matter issuing out of body orifices is polluting – pus, urine, sweat, saliva, nasal mucus, for example. This is the context in which breastmilk is perceived as an unclean secretion which, especially as it streams out unbidden and appears when socially inconvenient, is a waste product that has to be cleaned away. Other fluids that are specifically female – menstrual blood, lochia, amniotic fluid – are offensive too. In many societies they are not only polluting, but dangerous, and threaten male virility.

From puberty onwards, girls are educated to be secretive and ashamed about menstruation. Even when a girl is congratulated on becoming a woman, society's disgust about menstrual blood is communicated. All women's body products are to be hidden.

Breastfeeding and shame

For many women social pressures weigh more heavily than expert advice about breastfeeding. One of the most obvious of these is the general disapproval in western culture of breastfeeding in public. It is seen as an improper, even blatantly aggressive, act. While women's breasts are exposed widely in advertisements, on TV, in magazines, and some films, the lactating breast can cause revulsion.

This is most obvious in the context of food consumption. A woman who breastfeeds in a restaurant or anywhere where other people are eating is likely to meet with disapproval. A strict division must be maintained between food that enters the mouth and waste products that are excreted. Breastmilk is treated is a physical excretion. Revealing a lactating breast at the dinner table, for example, is like using a spittoon or a chamber pot.

Women breastfeed longer when they feel comfortable about doing it in front of other people. Yet breastfeeding openly is seen as a form of exhibitionism. Awareness of the social context in which breastfeeding takes place is a vital element in understanding how to support breastfeeding mothers.

If it is to take place outside the home, many women feel relaxed only when breastfeeding is disguised. So they offer a bottle, or resort to subterfuge. When a mother breastfeeds in public she often covers herself with a shawl or blanket and tries not to draw attention to herself. In some Arab cultures, where women's faces are veiled, mothers can breastfeed openly. In northern industrial cultures breastfeeding is made invisible.

In a UK publicity campaign for breastfeeding, the Department of Health produced photographs of fully clothed women with babies who are clearly not being breastfed, and for all we know may have been bottle-fed. There was one photograph of a father and baby in which his hairy chest was exposed. He was the only person in skin contact with a baby. It is not immodest for a man holding a baby to reveal his breasts. But it is for a woman. The concept of modesty is central whenever women avoid breastfeeding in front of other people.[18]

Being 'immodest' always involves an audience. Neither modesty nor immodesty exist in social isolation. When a woman is being immodest she displays to an audience. Embarrassment is an expression of the social interchange between the observed and the observer in an act that is considered shameful. This may be unilateral: a woman who is confident that she is doing the right thing can breastfeed openly without embarrassment (although she will probably need pluck and determination). An observer may actually approve of open breastfeeding, although the mother, aware of being noticed, still feels embarrassment.

A woman may be embarrassed when she accidentally draws attention to herself as lactating. This happens if, for example, she has expressed her milk and is presenting it to the baby in a bottle, but the baby snuggles up to her breast and roots for the nipple. Observers may also be embarrassed on seeing this.

But it is not only exhibition of the breasts that is considered immodest. Awareness that the baby is suckling, and enjoying it, may also threaten the

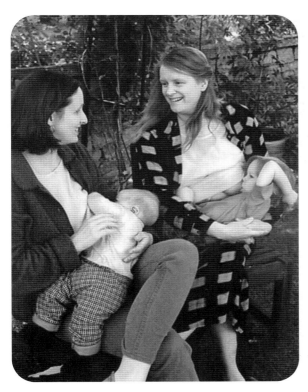

Friends enjoy breastfeeding a 6-month-old and a 2-year-old in the garden

woman's modesty and embarrass both her and those watching. Some babies are quiet feeders. Others display their pleasure with gusto, reaching out to touch and hold the breast, guzzling, slurping, lip-smacking, and coming off the breast for a bit, only to return like a salmon capturing a fly. This pleasure may be perceived as lascivious, and the mother as colluding in it. They are an out-of-control couple who fail to conform to normal standards of decency.

When either mother or child clearly enjoy breastfeeding it attracts critical attention. A woman is expected to fill a baby up with the same kind of detachment that she might have while pouring a cup of coffee. Any emotional element in breastfeeding is taboo.

If she has difficulty in getting a baby latched on and the baby seems to fight the breast, this also causes her acute embarrassment. It is not just that she is exhibiting her failure to mother. The conflict becomes a display of passion.

To keep breastfeeding disguised, not only must the breast be hidden, but the baby's behaviour must be kept muted, so that no one is aware of the act.

A woman may be exonerated of exhibitionism if she is breastfeeding a young baby, but attract critical attention and distaste when she breastfeeds an older child. In the first 3 or 4 months a baby is perceived as passive and receptive, not active and seeking. The indication is that it is all right to pour milk into an inert bundle wrapped in a shawl, but that there is something unhealthy about satisfying an older child's hunger for the breast.

Americans tend to be more uptight about nursing in public than Europeans. I have encountered this at first hand when negotiating with publishers over the photographs on the jackets of my books on breastfeeding. Publishers in Britain, Germany and Italy expect to have a photograph of a breastfeeding mother and baby on the book jacket. A New York publisher presented me with a cover photograph in which the nipples had been air-brushed out. When I objected, they substituted one of a baby with a frilled bonnet and lacy dress that hid the mother's breast entirely. The editor protested that she would love to show a baby really breastfeeding, but it was not possible in the USA. For many Americans, nursing a baby so that it is witnessed by other people is an act of sexual exhibitionism. Special nursing clothing is marketed, which has hidden plackets, seams and zips that enable breastfeeding to take place surreptitiously.

In England, breastfeeding in public can be awkward. It may be considered crude, exhibitionist or flamboyantly feminist. Scotland is ahead of the rest of the UK in passing a law (2004) under which businesses and public institutions are fined if they prevent women from breastfeeding openly. Bars, shops and restaurants have to accept breastfeeding.

Breastfeeding is declining even in Mediterranean cultures. Traditionally, a woman's virtue is defended aggressively by the male members of the family. They perceive other men as marauders who destroy modesty and thereby dishonour the whole family. Today bottle-feeding, because it eliminates display of the breasts, helps to protect women, and their male owners, against such attack. Women's breasts are considered their husbands' possessions. The man decides what is done with them and to whom they can be shown.

Shame and disgust about breastfeeding are closely connected to the view of a woman's body as male property. It is a concept that can only be understood in the context of a social analysis of gender relations. It turns out that men are the ultimate arbiters about what we do with our breasts.

References

1. Preston SH, Haines MR 1991 Fatal years: child mortality in late nineteenth-century America. Princeton, NJ: Princeton University Press

2. Wolf JH 2003 Low breastfeeding rates and public health in the United States. American Journal of Public Health 93(12):2000–2010

3. Freed GL, Clark SJ, Sorenson J, et al 1995 National assessment of physicians' breast-feeding knowledge, attitudes, training and experience. JAMA 273:472–476

4. Hamlyn B, Brooker S, Oleinikova K, et al 2002 Infant feeding 2000. London: Stationery Office

5. Declercq ER, Sakala C, Corry MP, et al 2002 Listening to mothers: report of the first national US survey of women's childbearing experiences. New York: Maternity Center Association

6. Graffy J, Taylor J, Williams A, et al 2004 Randomised controlled trial of support from volunteer counsellors for mothers considering breastfeeding. BMJ 328(7430):26

7. Thompson M, Westreich R 2000 Restriction of mother–infant contact in the immediate post-natal period. In: Enkin M, Keirse M, Renfrew M, et al (eds) A guide

to effective care in pregnancy and childbirth, 3rd edn. Oxford: Oxford University Press, pp 429–430

8. Kroeger M 2004 Impact of birthing practices on breastfeeding: protecting the mother and baby continuum. Sudbury, MA: Jones and Bartlett

9. Riordan J, Gross A, Angeron J, et al 2000 The effect of labor pain relief medication on neonatal suckling and breastfeeding duration. Journal of Human Lactation 16(1):7–12

10. Righard L, Alade MO 1990 Effect of delivery room routines on success of first breast-feed. Lancet 336(8723):1105–1107

11. Matthiesen AS, Ransjo-Arvidson AB, Nissen E, et al 2001 Postpartum maternal oxytocin release by newborns: effects of infant hand massages and suckling. Birth 28(1):13–19

12. Baumgarder DJ, Muehl P, Fisher M, et al 2003 Effect of labor epidural anesthesia on breast-feeding of healthy full-term newborns delivered vaginally. Journal of the American Board of Family Practice 16(1):7–13

13. Smith L 2004 Physics, forces and mechanical effects of birth on breastfeeding. In: Kroeger M (ed) Impact of birthing practices on breastfeeding: protecting the mother and baby continuum. Sudbury, MA: Jones and Bartlett, pp 119–145

14. Hall RT, Mercer AM, Teasley SL, et al 2002 A breast-feeding assessment score to evaluate the risk for cessation of breast-feeding by 7 to 10 days of age. Journal of Pediatrics 141(5):659–664

15. Kitzinger S 1983 Women's experience of sex. London: Dorling Kindersley

16. Douglas M 1966 Purity and danger. London: Routledge

17. Kegan P 1973 Natural symbols. London: Penguin

18. Moran M 1999 Analysis and application of the concept of modesty in breastfeeding. Journal of Perinatal Education 8(4):1

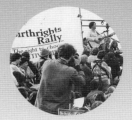

6
Birth education: from pedagogy to politics

The important thing is that whatever kind of birth she has a woman should be able to look back on it feeling positive about the way she coped, and start out on motherhood with self-confidence.

To present all births as the best possible is to manipulate reality and distort experience. Moreover, concentrating exclusively on experience at the personal level is a way to avoid having to challenge the medical system. Childbirth educators have a responsibility to address the political issues that underlie traumatic birth experiences.

The above two contrasting views of childbirth education are both my own, and both express how I feel – they are not the opinions of two different women. For this is the inner conflict many of us face as we try to give emotional support to individuals, and at the same time acknowledge that we must work to change the social conditions in which women are forced to give birth. I do not pretend that I have solved this conflict in my own mind. It is also a conflict that divides the childbirth movement: listening and teaching skills versus outspoken criticism and demands for change; individual counselling versus political activism.

The best birth educators are far more than instructors. They are sensitively aware of the emotional needs of women and their families, and share with each the journey to birth. This is the psychophysical journey as a new life enters the world, and the often stressful transition to parenthood that extends well into the year after.

My own conviction is that it is also our responsibility to be advocates for women in the struggle to reclaim childbirth. The politics of birth should be central to the work of birth organisations.

When a woman is unhappy about her experience, it is tempting to offer psychological explanations – to see her as having 'unrealistic expectations' and failing to 'adjust'. This is how traumatic experiences are often explained away by obstetric professionals. The woman herself is blamed. Birth organisations sometimes unwittingly collude with this by preparing women to maintain control over their behaviour and to adapt to interventions with good grace. Anger must be suppressed, and the resulting depression is treated as a personal psychological problem.

I believe that we must acknowledge anger, and use it constructively to help other women. When a woman has been traumatised by the experience of birth, the first task of the childbirth educator is to be with her in her pain, to be there to listen, accept and understand. But we have to go beyond this. We need to be able to redefine her problems in political terms.

At one level, the politics of birth entail bridge-building with hospital staff and administrators, supporting those doctors and midwives who give woman-centred care, and evolving practical strategies for improving the birth environment. But it also means that we have to protest against the violence that is done to women who are most vulnerable: the poor, the educationally disadvantaged, women of ethnic minorities, women categorised as high risk, those who cannot articulate their wishes and anxieties, and any woman who fears for her baby and is therefore easily persuaded to submit. We have a responsibility to resist institutionally sanctioned sexual abuse in the form of the rushed second stage, with barked commands to push, and routine incision of the woman's sexual organs. Still, in many countries, there are 90% episiotomy rates – a technological culture's way of female genital mutilation.

Rocking the boat

This philosophy used to get me into trouble regularly with the National Childbirth Trust (NCT). This is the organisation responsible for bravely introducing birth education into Britain in the 1950s, and today is still the most important body to train birth educators, breastfeeding counsellors and postnatal supporters, and to present childbearing women's concerns to government. I have supported and worked with the NCT from its beginning. Its greatest successes, however, have always been achieved through the energy of committed individuals, not committees, and not administrative policy. In fact, in the past these have often marginalised the individuals who could give most.

I had just had my first baby in France when the NCT was formed. My husband, Uwe, was in the diplomatic corps, and we came back to England when my daughter was 6 weeks old. It had been a wonderful home birth. The NCT launched an appeal for women to show pregnant women how to breathe and relax for labour. I ran groups, the first couples' classes in the UK, in our cottage outside Oxford. They were rather different from other antenatal classes of that time. Not only were partners present, but there was discussion about emotions and changing relationships. Because I was a social anthropologist, I wanted to look at the values in our birth culture, too, comparing them with those in other cultures. I never did believe in the exercise approach – selectively toning and stretching muscles and approaching birth as a gymnastic performance. Or, at least, I did not think it was enough to make birth joyful. These groups became very popular. People went to great effort to attend – one man wheeled his very pregnant wife in a large old-fashioned pram 5 miles from another village.

The NCT sprang from the philosophy of Grantly Dick-Read. In *Natural Childbirth*,[1] the book which later became *Childbirth Without Fear*,[2] he wrote that preparation for birth enabled a woman to sit and wait patiently for her baby and would 'beautify the maternal consciousness'. Natural birth would develop the innate 'feminine' qualities of patience, sensitivity and understanding, and enhance a marriage. He told the reader how to behave following birth, too. She should show 'a little more tenderness to her husband' in order to 'strengthen the bond of affection between them'. It sounded as if a new mother had a lot on her plate – not one baby to look after, but two!

This was the dominant ethos until psychoprophylaxis, which came from Russia via France, suddenly changed the purpose and style of birth education. The pregnant woman became a 'parturient' conditioned to jump through the flaming hoop of labour, so highly trained that every muscle was toned, and her mind a white blaze of determination. She was instructed to make an unwavering commitment to succeed at what was claimed to be 'painless' childbirth, achieved through breathing drills and distraction techniques. Women with 'intellectual conceit' – those who asked too many questions and did not have complete faith in the techniques – were certain to fail. Dr Fernand Lamaze claimed that working-class women who believed and obeyed what they were taught were much more successful.[3] Lamaze listed his results over 3½ years at the Clinique des Metallurgistes: 18.43% 'excellent' and 4.76% 'complete failure', the evidence for which was restlessness and screams. Women who suffered were themselves responsible, because they harboured doubts or had not practised sufficiently.[3]

When this method was first promoted in Britain by Erna Wright at the end of the 1960s, she introduced military metaphors. Labour became 'B-day' – a direct analogy with 'D-day', the landing of allied troops on the Continent in the Second World War. Birth became an athletic performance and women were treated like Pavlovian dogs conditioned to salivate at the sound of a bell.

For both Dick-Read and Lamaze, the issue was 'a woman's control over her own body rather her control over what other people are doing to it'. 'Far from explicitly challenging medical power … the NCT appealed to doctors' paternalism, asking them to be more indulgent of women at a time of particular vulnerability … It was a logical consequence of the Trust's "non-threatening" stance that it should present the inhumanity of the obstetric services as the unfortunate side-product of misunderstandings rather than the consequence of any conflict of interest or power-imbalance'.[4] Individual women could only hope to change things by being charming and tactful. Without radical change in the medical system, education for childbirth imposes a burden on women to put on a performance. They have to demonstrate that they can succeed.

Back in England I had given birth to twins, and had three babies under two. I planned to have them at home if everything was straightforward, but booked a hospital bed just in case. In fact, labour lasted 1½ hours from the first signs, and if I had attempted to get to hospital they would probably have been born in a lay-by on the A40. Uwe photographed everything, including me dancing (on a table for some reason) just before it all started, smiling as a head was born, and babies suckling. This at a time when women in birth photographs were commonly shown with their faces blacked out, or wearing masks. The twins were born on a Sunday, and on Thursday my class turned up to find the bump gone and two babies waiting to greet them. I joined the headquarters' NCT committee and used to travel by train to London with the babies head to toe in a carry-cot. Then two more babies came, and I had four under five and five under seven.

In those days it was difficult for pregnant women to find antenatal classes that were not didactic. You relaxed, breathed and received a large dose of reassurance, or practised conditioning exercises that trained you to react automatically to signals, and that was it. In many classes partners were still not invited to attend, except for a special 'fathers' evening'. In hospital classes a physiotherapist taught exercises, a midwife explained how the maternity unit worked, and an anaesthetist described the pain-relieving drugs that were on offer. The expectant mother was approached as a patient, not a woman in relationships with other people who were significant to her, and bringing with her experiences that might affect how she coped with childbirth. The social context in which we experience pregnancy, birth and motherhood was not explored.

The women who sought out NCT classes were, on the whole, comfortably off, middle class and white. Most

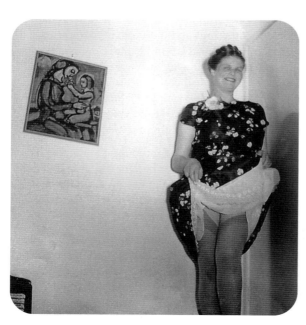

Sheila dances on a table, looking forward to her twins – born 36 hours later

couples were married. Single mothers were rare. Lesbians were unheard of. The NCT was looking for teachers who would fit snugly into that same pattern. Although it was a radical organisation, its teachers were expected to conform to the methods of the established leaders either of 'natural childbirth' or psychoprophylaxis.

I believed it was important to create a really good system to educate our NCT teachers. We developed teacher training based on the Oxford tutorial system, where individuals and small groups met with a tutor in a one-to-one continuing relationship. I devised essay topics, practical guidelines, exam questions and teaching observation. I hoped that our students would ask searching questions and challenge prejudices, and find the course exciting and mind expanding. Even so, as a tutor I discovered that a student who did not toe the line in terms of beliefs and life-style was likely to be rejected, or told that she was not yet quite 'ready'.

When my fourth baby was born she was waking at 5 a.m. for a breastfeed, and that had become my writing time. My first book, *The Experience of Childbirth*, broke new ground. Rather than being about breathing drills, which the then fashionable psychoprophylaxis advocated, it focused on the woman's total experience.

As time went on, the language I used changed. I deleted many words and phrases progressively over the years; references to 'old wives' tales', for example. Now I value the stories handed down from mother to daughter, and my real suspicion is more likely to be about 'obstetricians' tales'. I also wrote of 'the quality of the marriage relationship', and stated that 'our abilities as good mothers and fathers – and our families too – cannot be viewed in isolation, apart from the sum total – the interaction and fusing of personalities – which makes up the marriage'. Today I would not assume that there was a marriage, or a man.

I went on to write 24 other books, published in 20 languages, exploring different aspects of birth, the transition to motherhood, and female sexuality. One book that some in the NCT found threatening in the late 1970s was *The Good Birth Guide*.[5]

This was a report of women's experiences of antenatal, intrapartum and postnatal care, hospital by hospital all over Britain. It was rather like a restaurant guide, with recommendations for changes. Branches Forum, the nationwide meeting of NCT representatives, passed a vote of censure by an overwhelming majority, and I was reprimanded and warned that the book would damage relationships with hospitals that branches and teachers had been cultivating carefully for years. The administration also requested me not to refer to the NCT in media interviews. (Paradoxically, a few years later they wrote asking why when interviewed I never mentioned the organisation.)

The Good Birth Guide,[5] and *The New Good Birth Guide*[6] that updated it 5 years later, received extensive publicity. Thousands of women wrote to me about their birth experiences, and many obstetricians, paediatricians, midwives, and hospital administrators wrote to me of constructive changes they were making in response to the criticism. In the Introduction, I stated that much of the technology used in obstetrics at that time had become a routine part of clinical practice without adequate research and without strong evidence of its advantages. Moreover, many hospital rites were taken for granted by members of staff and performed as a matter of course, so that to question them seemed almost insulting.

It is the same today. Women in labour usually do not want to be thought 'rude' or aggressive, and as a result when they feel trapped in situations which are entirely out of their control, on territory over which power is exercised by professionals, they become passive and placating. Sometimes they are frightened into obedience because they fear that non-compliance will result in worse things being done to them or their babies. Change does not come, or does not come for enough women, when an expectant mother has a quiet talk with the obstetrician, but only when there is open and public protest. There is a place for quiet talks, but we need more than that if our culture of birth is to see any radical transformation.

This was strong stuff for those times. It is understandable that any consumer organisation eager to establish its credentials with the medical system, hoping to effect change by polite persuasion and tactful negotiation with those in power, should be anxious when an individual or subgroup within it seems to be rocking the carefully steered boat.

Janet Balaskas, who was one of my students training to be an NCT teacher, was asked to leave the course because her methods of getting women upright for birth were 'unproven' and considered too 'radical'. In her books on active birth[7] she captured images of women giving birth in upright positions, which shocked

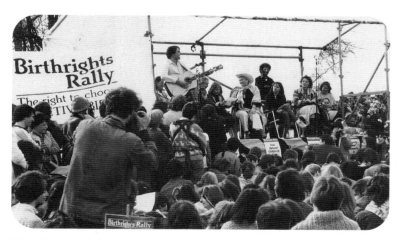

Five thousand parents, midwives and others protest at women being made to lie down during childbirth, 1982
(Reproduced with permission of Anthea Sieveking)

many people. She went on to found the Active Birth Movement, which has spread throughout the world.

The NCT acknowledged that the issue of home birth was important, and hosted a regular lunch group that I ran with professionals from different backgrounds – general practice, midwifery, psychiatry, psychotherapy, paediatrics and health economics – to examine home birth in depth. This resulted in a book that I co-edited with a distinguished Professor of Paediatrics, John Davis, called *The Place of Birth*.[8]

But the softly, softly approach was largely ineffective in changing obstetric practice, as increasingly intrusive technology and cumulative interventions established control over childbirth. Many positive changes were made too, but these came from outside the medical system. They were stimulated when women took matters into their own hands by changing hospitals or caregivers, and writing letters of complaint, when they joined together to demonstrate publicly and used the media to present their case, and when they chose home birth, declined interventions, and refused to act like well-behaved little girls who want to please teacher. Occasionally (although this is considered bad form in Britain), they even turned to litigation.

The NCT remained nervous of what its teachers and student teachers might be getting up to. As a result, some skilled and perceptive birth educators left. They were unable to explore new ways of teaching within it, felt frustrated by what seemed to them its slowly chugging bureaucracy, or believed that it was becoming too establishment oriented.

Matters came to a head in 1992, when the NCT Council decided to forbid childbirth educators to attend births. It feared conflicts with hospital staff and possible legal problems. But the teachers and the NCT tutors who trained them rebelled, and threatened to leave *en masse* and form their own organisation. In 1993 a newly elected Council decided that teachers could attend births at the invitation of the woman, and that the NCT would take out insurance to cover legal liability.

Meeting the challenge

Organisations are enriched when they tolerate and, indeed, welcome 'ginger' groups within their structure. They can benefit from their enthusiasm, their searching questions, and the articulation of new ideas. An organisation that cannot accommodate experiment is bound to atrophy or to be sucked into the establishment.

The challenge is to develop strategies that will improve the environment of birth for women everywhere, give women a voice, and link them powerfully together to ensure that the changes for which they are striving find practical expression. If that is 'rocking the boat', it is an essential part of our task.

The NCT has developed so that today it is politically active, working to correct the imbalance of power between professional care-providers and women giving birth, to educate those in the professions, and to ensure that positive government policies are translated into practice.

Already, in the last decade of the 20th century, the NCT was becoming more politically aware. In 1992 it lobbied and gave evidence to the Health Select Committee Enquiry into the maternity services, which produced a radical report led by the unlikely partnership of the Conservative MP Nicholas Winterton and the Labour MP Audrey Wise, an outspoken warrior for women's rights and birth issues. The Conservative Government had to reply to this report, and Eileen Hutton, NCT President, served on the Department of Health Committee that developed *Changing Childbirth*.[9] This document became government policy in 1993, advocating woman-centred care, with choice, control and continuity of care for all women.

The report challenged what it called the 'unproven assumption' that a hospital, by definition, provides optimal care for mothers and babies. In fact, it stated that 'the experience of the hospital environment too often deters women from asserting control over their own bodies and too often leaves them feeling that, in retrospect, they have not had the best labour and delivery they could have hoped for'. Women wanted choice as to the place of birth and carer. Fragmented care is dangerous. Home birth is a safe option, and women should be supported when they choose home birth. There must be a new professional role for midwives, together with midwifery-managed maternity units. 'We should move as rapidly as possible towards a situation in which midwives ... take full responsibility for the women who are under their care'.

When the Labour Government came to power, improving public health was a major part of its policies. The NCT took advantage of this and, at an open meeting in the House of Commons, the NCT and the Maternity Alliance stressed that the quality of birth is a vital element in public health. The message is that maternity care is not exclusively a woman's issue, but has life-long effects, for each individual and family, and for society as a whole. With this, the NCT underwent a metamorphosis from an organisation of childbirth educators and mainly middle-class mothers to one that speaks for all women and families. It now studies the government agenda and works out specific campaigns both to shape and develop that agenda and to coordinate action with consumer and professional organisations to improve care. It has researched women's access to information and support, for example, and revealed that young and ethnic minority parents have an urgent need for more open information and one-to-one support.

In 2000 the NCT set up a Maternity Care Working Party and an All-Party Parliamentary Group (APPG) to bring health professionals, parliamentarians, academics and consumer groups together, and explore with MPs how the recommendations in the document *Changing Childbirth*[9] could be put into action. At a recent count the APPG had 130 parliamentary members.

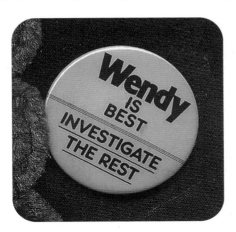

Out on the streets protesting in 1985, when obstetrician Wendy Savage was suspended from practice for respecting women's wishes

The NCT also began to do research into women's experiences of birth. This was new. When I undertook research into experiences of antenatal care, induction of labour, episiotomy and suturing of the perineum, epidurals and home birth in the 1970s and 1980s, the NCT published the results as reports or booklets, but I did the work independently, and without funding. It is very different now.

Another step forward in campaigning was establishing an effective press office to communicate with the media and keep birth issues centre stage, through questionnaires and surveys published in parenting magazines, and widely publicised. Multidisciplinary conferences and reports were organised, together with surveys that were often collaboratively carried out with magazines to fuel the debates by injecting new evidence.

Mary Newburn, the Policy Officer of the NCT, observed a 'sea change' with the appointment of Belinda Phipps, formerly a manager in the National Health Service (NHS), who understands how the NHS works and has introduced sharply focused strategic thinking. With a professional manager at its helm, the NCT became streetwise.

The NCT identified key figures in professional organisations who had influence with their peers. One result is that in 2001 the Royal College of Obstetricians and Gynaecologists (RCOG), Royal College of Midwives (RCM) and NCT jointly published *Modernising Maternity Care*.[10] This publication established benchmarks for a quality maternity service, asked Primary Care Trusts 'How do you stand?', and guided them on how to evaluate their own services.

The Maternity Care Working Party organised meetings on domestic violence, mental health and breastfeeding, and three successful conferences on what can be done to reduce the rising caesarean section rate. Half of all senior obstetricians consider these rates to be too high in their own hospitals.[11] This implies that the other half think that they are just right, or not high enough. One of these obstetricians (who shall be nameless and is now retired) wrote to a national newspaper, saying: 'I would advise them [women] that, soon after conception, they should book their caesarean section with epidural or spinal analgesia'.

But the tide is flowing in the opposite direction. Lesley Page, Head of Midwifery and Professor at Guy's and St. Thomas's, and Specialist Advisor to the House of

Commons Committee on Maternity Care, points out that in the USA midwifery has come from the counter-culture, whereas in the UK it is mainstream. The NHS would collapse without midwives. When midwives and consumers work together they speak with a powerful voice, and Parliament cannot ignore it.

In 2003 the APPG sent a letter to every maternity unit in England inviting it to compete for two awards, to be presented at the House of Commons by the Health Minister. One was the Increasing Normal Births Award and the other was the Most Improved Home Birth Rate Award. The letter went on to say: 'We would like you to look at your figures from April 2002 until now, and compare them with statistics in the previous two financial years. We want to hear from you if you feel efforts you are making to increase the numbers of normal births or improve home birth rates have been successful this year'. There is an additional note: 'Although the definition of a "normal" birth is one of much debate, for the purposes of these awards, we are defining "normal" as birth that starts, progresses and concludes spontaneously and one where the woman does not have anaesthesia or an episiotomy'.

For many women the NCT has served as a source for canalising energy, sharing ideas with other women, developing skills and working for change. For me it was never about coffee mornings. It was women working to reclaim childbirth as an exultant personal experience, rather than a medical event, and striving together for social revolution. The goal of normal birth for most women is one that the NCT, together with the two major Royal Colleges, is strenuously pursuing now. In childbirth it is not enough to aim to reduce the caesarean rate, not enough to ensure that all women have access to the information they need and get the same high-quality care. The challenge is for all obstetricians and midwives to respect the physiology of labour, and to acquire the understanding and skills to enable the vast majority of women to give birth normally.[6]

References

1. Dick-Read G 1933 Natural childbirth. London: Heinemann
2. Dick-Read G 1960 Childbirth without fear. London: Heinemann
3. Lamaze F 1956 Accouchement sans douleur. Paris: La Faradole
4. Kitzinger J 1990 Strategies of the early childbirth movement – a case study of the National Childbirth Trust. In: Garcia J, Kilpatrick R, Richards M (eds) The politics of maternity care. Oxford: Clarendon Press, pp 92–115
5. Kitzinger S 1979 The good birth guide. London: Fontana Paperbacks
6. Kitzinger S 1983 The new good birth guide. London: Penguin Books
7. Balaskas J 1991 New active birth. London: Thorsons
8. Kitzinger S, Davis J (ed) 1978 The place of birth. Oxford: Oxford University Press
9. Department of Health 1993 Changing childbirth. London: HMSO
10. Maternity Care Working Party 2001 Modernising maternity care: a commissioning toolkit for Primary Care Trusts in England. London: RCM/RCOG/NCT. Available at:

http://www.nctpregnancyandchildcare.com/nct-online/ModernisingMaternityCare.htm (accessed November 2004)

11. Thomas J, Paranjothy S 2001 Royal College of Obstetricians and Gynaecologists Clinical Effectiveness Support Unit. National sentinel caesarean section audit report. London: RCOG Press. Available at: http://www.rcog.org.uk/resources/public/nscs_audit.pdf (accessed November 2004)

7

The language of birth

Language expresses the way we think. It is also *shapes* the way we think. Language can *make* reality as well as reflect it. Think how the concept of the 'elderly primagravida' may dictate professional action in terms of potential illness and proposed treatment. Medical language affects not only the kind of care we receive, but also how we think about and experience our bodies.

The language of birth is rich with clues to its social meaning in any culture. In northern technocratic cultures medical language still dominates and constricts perception of the birth process, and obstetric practice assumes that labour and delivery are the results of an equation between 'the pelvis', 'the powers' and 'the passenger', with the mother rendered more or less invisible, whereas uterine contractility and cervical dilatation are often discussed as if they occurred on a laboratory bench rather than in a woman's body. Yet language in midwifery and birth education has been changing.

When my first book, *The Experience of Childbirth*,[1] was first and serialised in a Sunday newspaper I heard from hundreds of women sharing their experiences. Many of them seemed to find a voice for the first time. That was the start of thousands of letters and phone calls, and later e-mails, pouring in from women from around the world. Women poured out their joy and anguish, their anger and their love, describing their births and telling me how hospitals, doctors and midwives needed to change.

Women had been silent because there was no way in which to express their feelings. The language to convey the powerful physical sensations and overwhelming emotions of birth had to be created. Birth was discussed only as 'pain', as if that were the sum total of what labour and birth are about. Opening your body to let new life into the world is much more than that and has always had multiple layers of meaning for a woman, and for everyone else involved.

When I wrote that book in February 1963, I was in a state of postnatal euphoria. My fourth child was newborn. Like the others, it had been a home birth – and she was in the bed beside me in a room scented with hyacinths, in our cottage outside Oxford. I decided that I wanted to write about the joy of birth, and help other women discover it.

Polly was waking at around five in the morning for a breastfeed and then lay contentedly on the bed gazing around at her new world. I started to write *The Experience of Childbirth*. Writing early in the morning, in the first light of dawn, has stayed a habit – a quiet, peaceful time when my mind is still rich with waking thoughts, ideas and phrases. That first draft took me 6 weeks. Then I read it through aloud (that was important, I think, because I wanted to speak to women in my own voice, not to harangue them, and not to be literary) and amended it over another few weeks.

Since the 1960s I have called for positive images of pregnancy and birth, and challenged women to create their own language of birth. Yet, not so long ago, I heard antenatal teachers talk about the cervix as 'the weakest part of the uterus', the fetal head 'hitting' the pelvic floor, contractions feeling like 'severe period pains or a bad attack of gastroenteritis' or 'being sick the wrong end' and the sensations of the second stage as 'rather like pushing a frozen chicken along'.

The challenge I faced was to create a language to convey the multifaceted sensations of labour and birth, physical and emotional, to find words for the rush of energy as contractions welled up and squeezed the uterus, and the power that built mountains was released in your body, for the feeling as the baby's head crowned as if in a ring of fire, and the birth passion. I have been criticised for discussing giving birth in terms of sex, as if I were imposing on women a kind of sexual performance, birth with orgasm. But for me birth was an intense psycho-sexual experience. This is not surprising, since both childbirth and lactation involve the same hormones as sexual arousal, and both are an expression of what is going on in the mind, not just the body.

A few years later, an American, Marjorie Karmel, wrote *Thank you, Dr Lamaze* – to my mind a sycophantic book extolling the benefits of his method of strict training in breathing and relaxation.[2] It was an enthusiastic instruction manual. If a woman obeyed Lamaze's teachings she 'should' have no pain. If she did feel pain, however, it was evidence that she had not conformed to the 'correct' number of huffs and puffs or did not hold her breath long enough when pushing, failed to practice assiduously, and lacked commitment.

The contrast between psychoprophylaxis and my psycho-social approach stimulated lively debate, and the contrast in the ways in which language was used was one of the most striking differences. This was important, because it indicated fundamentally conflicting beliefs about birth.

Birth speak – some comparisons

In France the buzzword for midwives today is *accompagnement*. The midwife is to 'accompany' the mother, a term which is also employed when a mother takes her small child to school. When I discussed the changing language of French birth education and midwifery with Dr Michel Odent, he suggested that it implied dependency. There is no word for midwifery in French. The *sage-femme* practices *obstetrics*, and the most popular journal for midwives is entitled *Les Dossiers de l'Obstetrique*. The official definition of the role of the midwife is as a medical professional 'with limited competency'. In France techniques in the management of birth, along with some very old skills, are given pompous names derived from words of Greek origin. Hypnosis is 'sophrology'. 'Haptonomy', from the Greek *haptos*, is the science of touch, and there is a method of *hapto-obstetrique*. Midwives attend courses on the phenomenology of haptonomy and phenomenology of communication. The singing together that was started at Pithiviers, in which pregnant women, couples and staff all joined, has now become validated as *psychophonie*, and throughout France midwives are offered seminars in the technique. While midwifery practice is represented by pretentious concepts like these, it is not valued.

In contrast, the Italians are much influenced by British approaches to education for birth, and they now incorporate English words such as 'bonding' and 'partner' into their language of birth. The big buzzwords for them are 'humanised' – this turns up in the titles of dozens of conferences and booklets – and *autiogestione*, self-management, for the birthing woman.

In Britain, mechanistic concepts of birth interlocked neatly with the technology epidemic of the 1970s. The pregnant patient was perceived as either 'cooperative', a 'defaulter' or a 'difficult patient' who required special skills of management. Psychology was brought in to control her and to facilitate communication.

It is often taken as a sign of progress that pregnant women today have been turned into 'consumers'. This is happening all over western Europe. The Clinique des Lilas outside Paris offers, with fine gastronomic overtones, *l'accouchement a la carte*. Concepts of 'choice' are centre-stream in maternity care. Just as when she goes to a supermarket, where she can choose between breakfast cereals, a woman who is expecting a baby selects the system of care she prefers and chooses between drugs for pain relief. But the way in which these choices are presented defines and limits them. She may believe that she has more choice than she does.

Obstetric metaphors and marketing

Obstetricians use a language about pregnancy and birth that is very different from the language women speak. Labour and birth may be described in terms of 'the 3 Ps': the Pelvis, the Powers and the Passenger. When doctors – and midwives too – talk about a pregnancy being 'high risk', a labour being 'prolonged', 'an inadequate pelvis' or diagnose an 'incompetent cervix' or 'failure to progress' –

but especially when they make off-the-cuff comments about a 'lazy uterus', a 'sloppy cervix' or a 'boggy fundus' – they present a view of the world, and the place of women in it, that imposes a certain set of values and assumes that they, as professionals, can step back and make judgements separate from the objects and systems they study.

Obstetric language is mechanistic; women's is experiential. The obstetric script presents a pregnant woman as an ambulant pelvis. If she is having her first baby she is 'an untried pelvis'. In childbirth she is a 'contracting uterus' and a 'dilating cervix'. If she has a 'scarred uterus' she may be allowed 'a trial of labour' and is likely to perceive this as a trial of her as a woman.

Obstetric textbooks often adopt the language of architecture, as if the woman's body were a construction site.[3] There is the 'pubic arch', the 'pelvic floor', the 'abdominal wall' and the 'birth canal'. Metaphors are taken from industry, too. The process of birth is treated as the automatic movement of a bulky object, as if a manufactured product is being pushed mechanically along a conveyor belt that is constantly at risk of breaking down. Management of labour consists of keeping the conveyor belt running. In Sweden, antenatal care is called 'prenatal control', implying the management of female patients in much the same way as managers control factory products rolling off the assembly line. Sometimes obstetric writing suggests a DIY hobby. For example, when induction fails: 'The cervix gives way reluctantly with the impression that it is being forced open, like a door with hinges rusted' or, perhaps, with model aeroplane enthusiasm: 'Lift-off never occurs'.[4]

Much obstetric language is about conflict. The baby struggles with the maternal body for survival and her pelvis is seen as an arena in which these battles are fought. Certainly there are unhappy women hating pregnancy, who think of the baby inside them as a tumour feeding on their strength, swelling, growing, until they feel the baby has become a monster. We acknowledge that this is emotionally pathological. But when obstetricians use similar concepts, we accept this as their normal way of thinking. The fetus is 'competing' with the woman for nutrients, threatening her as its head grows ever larger, until finally, during labour, it tears muscles and tissues, and as it is propelled down the birth canal it damages the bladder, urethra, anal sphincter and perineum in the process of forcing its way out.

Such sadomasochistic language is well established in obstetrics. Joseph DeLee was a master of it:

> Labour has been called, and is still believed by many to be, a normal function. It always strikes physicians as well as laymen as bizarre, to call labour an abnormal function, a disease, and yet it is a decidedly pathologic process. Everything, of course, depends on what we define as normal. If a woman falls on a pitchfork, and drives it through her perineum, we call that pathological – abnormal, but if a large baby is driven through the pelvic floor, we say that it is natural, and therefore normal. If a baby were to have its head caught in a door very lightly, but enough to cause cerebral hemorrhage, we would say that

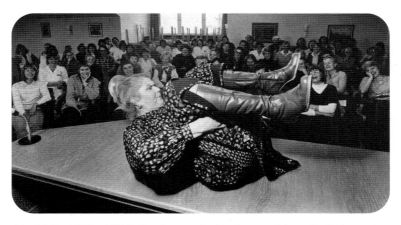

'Push! Push! Push!' Sheila demonstrates how *not* to get a baby out

> *it is decidedly pathologic, but when a baby's head is crushed against a tight pelvic floor, and a hemorrhage in the brain kills it, we call this normal ... In both cases, the cause of the damage, the fall on the pitchfork, and the crushing of the door, is pathogenic.*[5]

That is one view of women. Disaster in childbirth is our own fault because we should never have got up off all fours. He then moves from farm to fisheries:

> *I have often wondered whether Nature did not deliberately intend women should be used up in the process of reproduction, in a manner analogous to that of the salmon, which dies after spawning?*[5]

Today audio-visual aids may be used to emphasise that birth is dangerous and that a pregnant woman who spurns obstetric intervention does so at her peril. One German obstetrician actually sits patients down in front of a video of a simulated car crash, the head of a small child hitting the windscreen, to demonstrate what will happen at delivery if he does not perform an episiotomy.

Obstetric language employs metaphors of war and aggression: the 'aggressive management of ruptured membranes', the 'oxytocin challenge test', and the 'trigger factor' for labour, for example. In the Swedish language, to perform artificial rupture of the membranes is to 'explode' them, and in Swedish and Dutch the crowning of the baby's head is 'cutting through'.

In medical textbooks women are represented as headless, often cut up in little bits – a cervix here, a perineum there, an excised uterus over the page – and depicted as if they were simply a collection of bone, muscle and nerve fibres. Occasionally, humour intervenes and you get a complete woman in cartoon form. But she is ignorant, gross, a lump of meat with a pinhead at the far end. An anaesthetist, Felicity Reynolds,[6] believes that women should not be burdened with information about possible risks. Labour is like being on a plane. From the flightdeck the Captain – the obstetrician – makes an announcement: 'Welcome aboard this Boeing 747 flight to London. We should warn you that during this flight you may suffer hypoxia, dehydration, headache, backache, deep vein thrombosis, indigestion and constipation. In the event of disaster you may be burned to death, smashed to bits or slowly drowned'. Would it not be better, she implies, just to trust that he knows his job and let him get on with it?[6] She captions the cartoon: 'There is no need to spell out every conceivable risk'.

An obstetrician, Philip Steer, uses the language of neo-Darwinism to describe a battle between the baby and the mother: 'The scene is set for a competition between the fetus and the mother. It is inappropriate to see human labour as a harmonious process ... Labour should instead be seen as an imperfect solution to a complex problem'.[7] Steer believes that 'rather than indulging in reflex pleas to "return to the simplicity of nature" (which is often "red in tooth and claw"), we should be concentrating on making caesarean section even safer, researching ways to predict labours that will have an adverse outcome, and listening to what (properly informed) women want'. Steer sees birth in terms of the size of the female pelvis in relation to the size of the baby's head; because human beings have evolved big brains they often cannot get through the female pelvis without catastrophe. This ultra-Darwinism ignores the social and environmental aspects of birth. It reduces the whole process to a contest between the mother and the fetus.

With a little lateral thinking we might come to very different conclusions. We could ask, for example: 'What is there about obstetric methods of managing labour and about the birth environment that tends to make birth difficult and might contribute to the present high rates of caesarean section?'

In the late 1920s Professor Solly Zuckerman studied baboons in London Zoo and reported that they lived in a perpetual state of violence. On this foundation he created a theory of social behaviour which became very influential. Every baboon 'seemed to live in perpetual fear lest another animal stronger than itself would inhibit its activities'. The social order frequently collapsed into 'an anarchic mob, capable of orgies of wholesale carnage'.[8] Other researchers were unable to replicate his findings when working with baboons in the wild. It turned out that those in the zoo behaved like this because they were kept in captivity in a restricted space. In his ground-breaking book *Lifelines: Biology, Freedom, Determinism*, the biologist Steven Rose criticises 'the prevailing fashion for giving genetic explanations to account for many if not all aspects of the human social condition – from the social inequalities of race, gender and class to individual propensities such as sexual orientation, use of drugs or alcohol, or the failures of the homeless or psychologically distressed to survive effectively in modern society'.[9] This is the ideology of *biological determinism*, typified by the extrapolations of evolutionary theory that comprise much of what has become known as *sociobiology*. It is this kind of theory that has been incorporated into a plea for more caesarean sections.

This argument is often tied up with the concept of 'choice' and retailing. This was basic to the British Government document *Changing Childbirth*, published in 1993, that I talked about in Chapter 6.[10] This publication set the scene for a new policy of maternity care in England and Wales. 'Women should receive clear, unbiased advice and be able to choose where they would like their baby to be born. Their right to make that choice should be respected and every practical effort made to achieve the outcome that the woman believes is best for her baby and herself'. Phil Steer picked up on this, said that an increasing proportion of women are requesting caesarean section, affirmed that 'taking heed of women's views is fundamental to achieving a satisfied customer', and incorporated language drawn from marketing to justify elective caesareans. [7] The customer is always right, or at least, one who is 'properly informed'. The language of choice has been appropriated by obstetrics.

The language of rape

In fact, many women are desperately disappointed and feel cheated – even abused – by what they have gone through in childbirth. When women call me on the Birth Crisis helpline, time and time again I hear the same phrases:

'I wasn't allowed to ... I had to ... ', 'They spoke about me, "over" me, not to me', 'I wasn't a person any more ... just an object', 'a number and a case ... ', 'I was supposed to be a good girl and not make a fuss', 'The midwives never said hello ... there was no emotional support ... they were screaming at me, "Push! Push! Push!"', 'I couldn't move. They said that I had to lie on my back. When I moved it interfered with the print-out from the monitor', 'They didn't explain ... I don't know what happened or why. It is all a muddle', 'It felt like a "conveyor belt"'. They say they were like a 'fish on a slab', 'trussed up like an oven-ready turkey', 'a piece of meat'.

Women felt blamed, and often threatened: 'I was told I could kill my baby', 'It was my fault because I didn't push hard enough', 'He told me that if I didn't consent to a caesarean I could have a brain-damaged baby', 'Suddenly the room filled with people. There was a man with his head between my legs'. A woman whose baby died says she was told: 'You squeezed the life out of that baby'.

These women feel violated. They use the language of rape.

For them *pain* is not the central issue. The important thing is how they were treated, what people did to them – the relationships with their caregivers.

'Continuity' of care

'Continuity' is a buzzword in midwifery that often sounds more impressive than it is in practice. It may cast a positive glow around midwifery without meaning much. In a hospital where there was a written policy of one-to-one midwifery, video recording of 20 women through the first and second stages of labour revealed that 108 clinicians – midwives and doctors – came in and out of the room while they laboured (the greatest continuity came from registrars working on extended shifts). Of these 20 women, 14 had to cope with one shift change and three with two shift changes. Midwives sat and talked to mothers for only 15% of the time. No doctor ever sat down and had a conversation with a mother.[11] Decisions about treatment were often made outside the room, so that parents could not participate in the discussion.

In spite of all the lip-service about continuity, most women giving birth have fragmented care. This not only means that they are unable to form relationships with the professionals they encounter, but that it is emotionally unsatisfying for the midwives and doctors caring for them, too.

'Control' in childbirth

There is another aspect of choice that is important. It is usually claimed that good communication is bound to result in 'informed consent'. An equally valid outcome is 'informed refusal', particularly when women become aware of research evidence about electronic fetal monitoring (that it is not reliable), home and hospital birth (for women with no special risk factors home is safer), and induction of labour before 42 weeks (it leads to increased ventouse and forceps deliveries, and caesarean sections). In spite of lip-service to randomised controlled trials and emphasis on the importance of evidence-based medicine, compliance is perceived as a consequence of effective patient management. A psychologist working in a National Health Service maternity unit explained that good communication means that 'compliance and informed consent can be increased'.[12] While 'informed consent' echoes through the language of birth, 'informed refusal' is rarely tolerated.

There is one word, however, the meaning of which has changed dramatically. That is 'control'. When psychoprophylaxis was in fashion it implied self-control on the part of the woman who successfully applied the pain-prevention techniques she had learned in pregnancy. Velvoski, in his book on psychoprophylaxis, announced that 'labour should not hurt; must not hurt'.[13] And this because the woman was 'in control' and did not weakly give way to pain. In Moscow, an obstetrician boasted to me about the success of this training: 'The labour wards are silent now. The mothers make no sound'. That is one way of suppressing women.

Today 'control' is a vital element in 'empowering'. Often that is just sweet talk. But it should mean that a woman is free to obtain the information she needs to make her own decisions, and to control the environment for birth, and everything that is done to her and her baby.

To change our culture so that birth becomes woman-centred is a painfully slow and frustrating struggle. But the radical change in the meaning of the single word *control* is probably the biggest breakthrough that has been achieved in the language and thinking about birth.

Yet even that can be deceptive. When you go into a restaurant you may think 'I'll have the prawns or the Greek salad and then I'd like the truffle risotto'. In childbirth you can be in control of your environment. You can control what people do to you. You can breathe your way through contractions and move freely and rock your pelvis and shout and sing. But you can no more control birth than you can control the tides of the sea. Birth is at one with the creation of the world, the building of mountains, the sweep of the wind, the cycles of night and day, and the waxing and waning of the moon. When we talk about 'control' and 'birth plans' and the choices we have we need to use this metaphorical language too, the power of all our senses, and the language of drama and poetry. Then more women will emerge from childbirth triumphant and radiant with joy and fulfilment.

References

1. Kitzinger S 1962 The experience of childbirth. London: Victor Gollancz

2. Karmel M 1965 Thank you Dr Lamaze. New York: Dolphin Books

3. Martin E 1987 The woman in the body: a cultural analysis of reproduction. Boston: Beacon Press

4. O'Driscoll K, Meagher D 1980 Active management of labour. London: WB Saunders, p 158

5. DeLee JB 1920 The prophylactic forceps operation. Paper presented at 45th Annual Meeting of the American Gynecological Society, 24–26 May 1920. American Journal of Obstetrics and Gynaecology 1:24–44, 77–80

6. Reynolds F (ed) 1997 Pain relief in labour. London: BMJ Publishing, p 180

7. Steer P 1998 Caesarean section: an evolving procedure? British Journal of Obstetrics and Gynaecology 105:1052–1055

8. Russell C, Russell WMS 1968 Violence, monkeys and man. London: Macmillan

9. Rose S 1998 Lifelines: biology, freedom, determinism. London: Penguin, pp 1–7

10. Department of Health 1993 Changing childbirth. Part 1: Report of the Expert Maternity Group, vol 2. London: HMSO, p 25

11. Harris M 2002 An investigation of labour ward care to inform the design of a computerised decision support system for the management of childbirth. Unpublished doctoral thesis, University of Plymouth

12. Sherr L 1995 The psychology of pregnancy and childbirth. Oxford: Blackwell Science

13. Velvoski I, Platonov K, Ploticher V, Shugom E 1960 Painless childbirth through psychoprophylaxis. Moscow: Foreign Languages Publishing, p 225

8
Touch and its meanings

Touch is a way of giving and receiving information, not only about objects, but also about feelings. How, where, when and whom we touch is patterned by culture and is an expression of the relative status of each person involved and the social distance or proximity between them. Touch often conveys messages that we do not intend and of which we are not aware.

For any researcher of the birth environment, observation of touch and avoidance of touch is an important tool in understanding the meanings that birth has for the midwife, the obstetrician, the mother and the father.[1]

What can be learned from touch?

Touch is often talked about as invariably a good thing. After all, it entails making contact. It is one human being reaching out to another. But touch is not necessarily a good thing – it can also be threatening, coercive or abusive. In recording behaviour it helps to develop a code for touch alongside observation of speech and other interactions.

In the medical model of birth, touch is largely restricted to certain individuals with professional authority. The mother may not be able to touch herself below the waist. Her partner can kiss her, mop her brow, hold her hand, rub her back, but is not permitted to massage her perineum, introduce a finger into her vagina, or feel the baby's head as it crowns. Each participant in birth – the obstetrician, the midwife, the mother and the father – has rights over specific territory of the woman's body and is limited to certain kinds of touch, and no other.

A woman describing her labour said: 'I put my hand down because it hurt so much and I touched the part where the baby's head was coming out. The midwife snorted and said sarcastically, "What do you think you are doing? Do you intend to deliver the baby yourself then?" I felt ashamed. I shouldn't have touched myself down there'.

Ideas about appropriate touch vary with the birth culture. I was told by a witch doctor in South Africa that, among the Bushmen, if a birth is difficult a witch doctor is called who applies his or her lips to the woman's vulva and attempts to suck out the baby with a ventouse-like action. In South African pastoral tribes, if labour is long the midwife may try to encourage the baby to emerge by letting it 'smell the father's cows' and so realise how wealthy he is. She smears vaseline over the woman's perineum and inside the birth canal and then packs it with cow dung. It is, without question, a dangerous practice. In India and Africa the midwife may use her big toe pressed against the woman's anus to guide the baby's descent and, as the baby's head is about to crown, a toe to guard the perineum.

The language of touch

Diagnostic touch is used in all birth cultures. The Indian *dai* palpates the uterus to feel the *jee* or *jeevan* (life energy) and to diagnose presentation. In traditional birth cultures vaginal examination is rarely employed, whereas in the medical model it is performed at least every 2 hours in labour and every 10 minutes, or more frequently, in the second stage.

In the medical model of antenatal care, abdominal palpation is a routine part of midwifery screening throughout pregnancy and may be performed at every visit. Midwives may assume that it is reassuring for women. Yet it is often uncomfortable and can be painful and anxiety-arousing: 'They pull your knickers down and dig in'; 'I felt quite bruised afterwards'; 'Some of them have really long nails – one of them scratched me'.[2] Proposing a woman-centred approach, a midwife writes that now she always asks first: 'Would you like me to feel the baby?' and 'May I touch?'; 'I ask the woman if she would like to feel for herself, and take her hands so that together we feel the various parts of the baby. Partners and other children often get involved as well'.[2]

Regular vaginal examinations are a normal part of care during childbirth, and midwives may not perceive them as an intervention. They are intrusive, can be painful and may communicate anxiety and cause distress. 'Why does she need to keep on shoving her fingers in if everything's OK. Is something wrong?' The information these examinations offer is often important, but they may 'reinforce actual messages about women's powerlessness and imply that the woman's body cannot be trusted to work right'.[3] After looking at all the research evidence, Professor Murray Enkin concludes that 'repeated vaginal examinations are an intensive intervention of as yet unproven value'.[4]

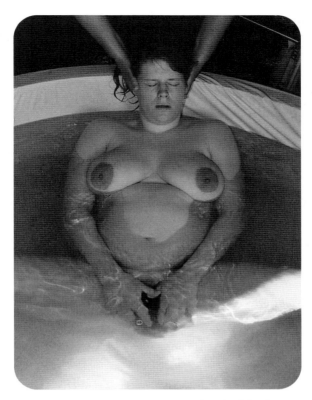

**The midwife cradles the mother's head while the
mother cradles her baby's head as it slides forward**

Experienced midwives working outside the medical model use touch in a very
sophisticated and sensitive way:

*I can anticipate a birth best when I concentrate on information that comes to
me through my hands down, tracing the path the baby will take, I feel smooth,
strong muscles and a baby who rides in a taut pouch. With experienced
birthers, I can close my eyes and feel the revelation of work done, of skin
that has stretched and reknit, of muscles that have spread and drawn back
together. I can feel tenacious parts and those that are more lax. I can
anticipate muscular dynamics. I can feel whether there is a good pool of
waters, whether the baby has sufficient mass, and how vital it is. I probe for
the baby's head or bottom riding above a pubic bone. Placing my right hand
on the hard, softball-like mass there and putting my left on the corresponding
ball just below a rib cage, I ask a woman to take a deep breath. As her
abdominal muscles relax, I can rock what is, most often, the baby's head. If it
is not a little free, this mass, I'd suspect it might be the baby's bottom I am
trying to wag and so reverse my manoeuvre. Later in pregnancy, I look for the*

69

head or bottom to slip deeper into the pelvic purse and get stodgy. When it's dropped out of reach, I can pretty much exclude placenta praevia, which means hemorrhage, and cord prolapse.[5]

In technocratic birth midwives seldom learn these skills. Diagnostic instruments are used and a fetal monitor or ultrasound scan replaces human contact.

Touch is often not only diagnostic but also *manipulative*. External version is used to turn the baby from breech to a cephalic presentation. In traditional birth cultures the midwife may rotate the baby from posterior to anterior with abdominal massage and, in Mexico, for example, hands are used to rock the pelvis in an action known as 'sifting'. The *partera* also massages the mother's legs to diagnose tension caused by the pressure of the baby's presenting part against her spine, and follows this with abdominal, low back, sacroiliac, foot, head and neck massage and manipulation.

An American midwife who works with the Amish people writes:

Sometimes I see swelling in the small of the back and know that the baby's head is ramming against a body ledge. I ask the woman to squat down and to grip her husband's hands or the end of the bed for balance. I drop down in back of her, slip my fingers around the wingtips of her pelvis, place my knee in the small of her back and press. The pelvis, like a bow, springs the baby's head off the shelf and lets it slide down onto the lower curve of backbone that will guide it out.[6]

Touch to *give comfort*, *release tension* and *ease pain* is offered generously in traditional birth cultures. Perineal and vaginal massage with oil is described in the Talmud. Midwives in South African pastoral tribes use beef fat to massage the perineum, and it was used in this way in Victorian England, too. In Thailand holy water is used for whole-body massage.

Comfort touch

This often consists simply of hand or shoulder holding, brushing the mother's hair, and kissing or cuddling her. In Mexico, the *partera* gives comfort touch, but there is also another woman, the *tendera*, whose main task is to hold and touch. In a medical model of birth the mother may never receive touch of this kind, or it is provided by a birth companion who is not part of the medical system. Diagnostic, manipulative and pain-relieving touch are combined in the actions of the Zulu midwife when she diagnoses a posterior presentation, firmly massages the mother's buttocks, and presses against and lifts her coccyx at the height of each contraction.

Today, in a medicalised system, when the mother has a partner or other companion, massage is often used to give comfort. It is taught to fathers in antenatal classes, partly to build up their confidence. A midwife who surveyed the birth experiences of 30 fathers concluded: 'Doing something seems more

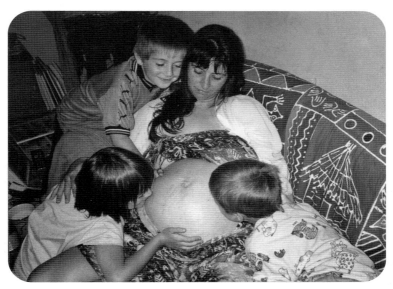

The other children feel the unborn baby in wonder

controlling than doing nothing'.[7] The same applies to midwives and obstetricians. Another midwife surveyed the birth experiences of 50 couples and showed that massage helped women cope with pain and enabled the partners to feel more involved. She suggests that: 'These massage techniques offer one way of overcoming the helplessness felt by many men when they are with women in labour'.[8]

Physically supporting touch merges with *comfort touch*. Helpers use their own bodies so that the mother can stand, sit, kneel or squat. Lap-sitting, with the mother crouched between the thighs of a helper, is common. In the past it was often used in Europe too, and among the early North American colonists.

I have coined the term the *blessing touch*, to represent touch that can draw on spiritual power. It communicates energy from the ancestor spirits, God or nature. Oils or holy water may be used, and it then becomes *anointing*. The effectiveness of this form of touch is rooted in the culture and relies on the mother and midwife sharing the same beliefs.

Restraining touch is used to ensure that the mother stays in one position, remains still during examinations and manipulations, and does not contaminate the 'sterile area'. It is frequently employed in medicalised birth.

A woman describing the way in which the second stage of labour was managed says: 'My legs were held up by a midwife and my husband. I felt so embarrassed, humiliated and useless that I couldn't even do this for myself'.

But the restraining touch becomes unnecessary as machines and obstetric equipment replace the human hand. The mother can be strapped into lithotomy stirrups and wrist-cuffs instead: 'I was trussed up like an oven-ready turkey'. Or an epidural can ensure that the woman is partially or completely immobilised. This tends to be how women prisoners are restrained once shackles are removed.

Restraining touch overlaps with *punitive touch*, when the mother is slapped or an examination is performed roughly.

Abusive touch

In a technocratic birth culture, women may describe how they were 'poked and prodded', 'mauled', even 'butchered'. Afterwards the woman is anxious, stressed, finds it difficult to concentrate, is hectically active, and may have panic attacks, nightmares and flashbacks to the birth: 'He rummaged me around', 'I was skewered'.

While it is acknowledged that rape is psychologically damaging, the woman who feels that she has been violated in childbirth is expected to be grateful to those who have saved her and her baby from disaster. This is a major element in post-traumatic stress following birth.

Understanding the message of touch

To understand the messages that health professionals and other helpers give women in childbirth we need to deconstruct the language of touch. More sensitive awareness of how we touch, and how touch is received, can help us understand what is being communicated over and above words. Touch is as important an element in the interaction between professional caregivers and women in childbirth as is spoken language, and because labour is an intensely physical process can have a powerful impact on women's whole experience of childbirth.

References

1. Kitzinger S 1997 Authoritative touch in childbirth: a cross-cultural approach. In: Davis-Floyd RE, Sargent CF (eds) Childbirth and authoritative knowledge. Berkeley, CA: University of California Press, pp 209–215

2. Olson K 2003 'Now just pop up here, dear'. Revisiting the art of antenatal abdominal palpation. In: Wickham S (ed) Midwifery best practice. Oxford: Books for Midwives

3. Bergstrom L, Roberts J, Skiliman L, et al 1992 'You'll feel me touching you, sweetie': vaginal examinations during the second stage of labor. Birth 19(1):10–18

4. Enkin M 1992 Do I do that? Do I really do that? Like that? [commentary]. Birth 19(1):19–20

5. Armstrong P, Feldman S 1990 A wise birth. New York: Morrow, p 49

6. Armstrong P, Feldman S 1990 A wise birth. New York: Morrow, p 50

7. Nolan M 1994 Caring for fathers in antenatal classes. Modern Midwife 4(2):25–28

8. Kimber L 2003 How did it feel to you? An informal survey of massage techniques in labour. In: Wickham S (ed) Midwifery best practice. Oxford: Books for Midwives

9
The caesarean epidemic

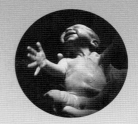

Caesarean section is promoted in the USA as a way of 'keeping your vagina honeymoon fresh'. It is sometimes referred to in the British press as 'the sunroof option', and is invariably treated as life-saving for the baby and a safeguard for the mother's health and sexuality. If you do not have a caesarean you risk your vagina getting flabby, your pelvic floor muscles collapsing, your bladder leaking – and losing your man.

A study of London obstetricians' views about caesarean section revealed that 31% of female obstetricians would want an elective caesarean, even if there were no special indications. This research was picked up by the media and hit the headlines. Of these female obstetricians, 88% feared perineal and bladder injury if they had a vaginal birth and 58% were concerned that vaginal birth might damage long-term sexual function.[1]

Subsequently an American survey showed that 46% of US obstetricians would also personally opt for caesarean section.[2] This built-in clinician bias is likely to affect the advice women are given and, in turn, the decisions they make.

Alan Brown, an Edinburgh consultant obstetrician, commented in a lecture at the Royal Society of Medicine that the research from which the London obstetricians drew their evidence was done in the early 1960s by a Liverpool obstetrician, Winnie Francis.[3,4] She revealed that urinary incontinence developed *antenatally* in 50% of primigravidae and 80% of multigravidae. Birth itself did not cause leakage unless significant cephalopelvic disproportion occurred or there was a difficult delivery, and incontinence was rare unless the anal sphincter was torn. With this in mind, Alan Brown said that, because the risk from vaginal birth is so small, he would try to dissuade any patient from choosing a caesarean, but would accept whichever decision a woman arrived at after counselling.[5]

Some obstetricians studiously ignore or brush aside impatiently the results of randomised controlled trials of caesarean birth. Professor Nick Fisk, at Queen Charlotte's Hospital in London, which has both high epidural and high caesarean rates, promotes them with enthusiasm. He was an author of the London survey of his colleagues' attitudes,[1] but says that, quite apart from this, more and more patients are demanding caesarean section. He predicts that rates will reach 50% in a few years, and says that an elective caesarean is very safe compared with driving a car. It is, he claims, the safest method of delivery for modern mothers and babies, and female obstetric staff and obstetricians' wives are booking caesareans as soon as they know they are pregnant. On TV he claimed that this is because of 'increasing maternal input into childbirth'. I am not sure what he means by this. Birth always entailed a great deal of 'maternal input'. Obstetricians could not produce babies without it. The debate about caesarean section, like the wider debate about screening procedures in pregnancy and active management of birth, is one about control over territory. The disputed territory is a woman's body.

An obstetrician at a private London hospital, the Portland, argued in the press that 'there are great advantages to having a caesarean. You can choose who is going to do the delivery. And it is marvellous for people who want the social convenience of knowing exactly when they are delivering ... It is a good option for women who are worried about pain and about possible bladder damage or sexual dysfunction'. He went on to claim that if a woman 'is older or it is to be her last pregnancy, an elective caesarean is a better option and less risk to the baby'. Then, astonishingly, he added with great honesty, 'There is an argument for caesareans when a doctor wants to protect himself against being sued by a patient, particularly in cases where there has been a difficult delivery before. There are also financial considerations. With a normal pregnancy and normal delivery, you can't claim off your health insurance policy unless it is a European or American one with higher premiums and less exclusions. But there is an inducement for the patient to opt for a caesarean if the insurance company will pay, because the whole process is then cheaper for the patient'.[6]

Other obstetricians are more temperate. I was surprised when an eminent gynaecologist, with whom I had publicly drawn swords about home birth and his policy of insisting that women deliver their babies in a supine position, stated in a radio discussion that he agreed with me and was 'ashamed' of what fellow obstetricians were saying in the press. There appears to be a divide between both some older and younger obstetricians and between those who concentrate on National Health Service (NHS) work and those doing private obstetrics. As in all other countries, those working outside the health service have much higher caesarean rates.

In Sweden the caesarean section rate declined from 12% in 1983, the highest rate it had ever reached there, to 10.8% in 1990. At the same time perinatal mortality rates were reduced by half.[7] Nordic countries are the only ones that have succeeded in keeping their caesarean rates from rising and where the rates did not exceed 14% through the 1990s.[8]

In Britain the caesarean rate was 4% in 1970, 10% in the early 1980s, 15% in 1994, and 16% in 1996. By the year 2000 it had risen to 21.5%. In July 1997 the Labour Secretary of State for Health, Frank Dobson, required NHS Trusts to audit caesarean rates for the first time. This was because finances were being drained from other areas of healthcare to cover the extra £750 ($1245) that each caesarean birth cost over a vaginal birth.

It is difficult to generalise about costs, as they depend on how services are organised in each area. In Torbay, where there is a highly efficient community-based system of care with an excellent ratio of one midwife for every 26 women, 75% of women have midwife-led care and there are some 230 home births a year. Lynne Leyshon, Head of Midwifery there, estimates that an elective caesarean costs twice as much as a hospital delivery without complications, and a home birth half as much as a hospital birth.[9]

Shrewsbury has a particularly low caesarean rate – 10.9%.[10] This is attributed mainly to the fact that almost one-third of pregnant women never see an obstetrician. Of those who have had a previous caesarean, 70% have a successful vaginal birth.[11]

Who has caesareans?

The rate of caesarean sections does not seem to match need, and there is a corresponding increase in the proportion of low birth weight and pre-term babies who require special care.[12]

Wherever women who are having normal births are treated as though they are at high risk and have overmanaged labours, the chances of ending up with a caesarean section are multiplied. That is one reason why the caesarean rate in Britain is twice that in The Netherlands, where a third of births take place at home and most women have total care from midwives.

The one-child family policy in China has contributed to the popularity of caesarean sections – 32% in the Shanghai area, for example. Women who are only allowed to have one child seek a 'quality baby' and a Professor of Obstetrics explained to me that his patients insist on caesareans because they are convinced they are safer than vaginal births. But how did women get this idea in the first place?

There are no national statistics for caesarean sections in India, but in the area around Madras the rate was 45% in 2000.[13] In countries such as India and Thailand, caesarean delivery is a symbol of high status.

On the other hand, over large parts of Africa, women who need caesareans cannot get them. The rate in west Africa is as low as 1.3%, although it has been estimated that up to 6.5% should have them.[14]

In all countries, women who give birth in private hospitals are at greatly increased risk of having surgery. Brazil has one of the highest rates of caesarean section in the world. There, over 90% of women in some private hospitals have caesareans. The rate as a whole was 72% in 2001. But even clinic patients have high caesarean rates – 34% in one of the poorest regions and 31% in the public sector generally.[15] It is sometimes claimed that this is because women 'demand' them. One study revealed that in a city in southern Brazil a high proportion of women 'expected' to deliver by caesarean section.[16] This is not the same as showing that women *want* them. Other studies make it clear that about 80% of women, regardless of whether they are private or clinic patients, prefer to give birth vaginally.[15, 17]

It has been suggested that 'scheduling caesarean sections is a way in which obstetricians accommodate their working and leisure time. Although caesareans are common among private patients, the trend for caesarean sections may have a knock-on effect on socially unprivileged women seeking what they perceive to be good healthcare during delivery'.[18] On the other hand, one reason why poor women with large families hope for a caesarean section is that it may be the only way to achieve effective birth control. They are offered tubal ligation together with the caesarean.[19] Women without regular access to contraception and those who submit to men because it is considered men's right to have sex when they want it, seek tubal ligation, and the only way to be certain of getting it is to deliver by caesarean. For all Brazilian women the obstetrician defines the situation so that women may be relieved and grateful when told they need a caesarean. In Chile, too, whereas approximately 70% of women with private care have caesareans, the rate of caesareans in the public sector is only about half that (25–30%).[20]

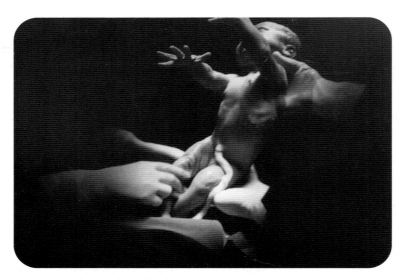

A mother's first sight of her baby born by caesarean

Continuous electronic fetal monitoring pushes up the caesarean rate. An essential element in the aggressive management of labour is the routine use of electronic fetal monitoring. The American College of Obstetricians and Gynecologists advised its members to stop routine electronic monitoring in 1995. Yet the use of such monitoring continues to soar in the USA (it was already used in 81% of all births in 1995),[21] and it is increasing in all European countries. Women often have a caesarean section simply because they are harpooned to monitors. These can give false readings, produce print-outs that are interpreted wrongly, and prevent the woman from adopting upright positions and moving freely. Randomised controlled trials comparing electronic fetal monitoring with intermittent auscultation show higher rates of caesarean sections in the electronically monitored groups.[22] Studies in the 1970s revealed that, when used without fetal blood sampling as well, monitoring increases the chance of caesarean section by an amazing 160%.[23]

But, as Nick Fisk points out, 'if you say to a woman that there's a 1% chance this may save the baby's life, she'll take it'.[24] Epidurals, especially given before 5 cm dilatation, can also have an effect of doubling the caesarean rate.[25] Women are grateful that their babies have been 'saved' by caesarean section, not realising that the way labour was managed, starting with induction, and followed by an intervention that screwed up the normal physiology of labour, resulted in caesarean section when the cervix did not dilate. The justification for caesarean delivery is usually 'failure to progress'. Some caesareans are obviously life-saving. Others are not. Yet the mother feels relief, and only later questions whether or not it was necessary.

Obstetricians often explain that the rise in caesareans is due to the threat of litigation. If something bad happens to a baby, it is safer to show that you did something rather than nothing, and deciding on a caesarean section is an obvious way to demonstrate concern. Nick Fisk is reported as saying: 'if you add up the risks, there is a one in 400 chance of brain damage or death if a baby is born vaginally. Elective caesareans or induced births obviate that',[9] and this is what he tells pregnant women.

Most multiple and breech babies are now delivered by caesarean section, although 'There is no clear evidence of benefit'.[26] The practice is likely to continue on the grounds that 'it's better to be safe than sorry!'

A major reason why the caesarean rate is shooting up is that obstetricians have become de-skilled. Older, experienced obstetricians know how to deliver a breech vaginally. Younger, less experienced obstetricians prefer to do a caesarean section. Older, experienced obstetricians can also perform external cephalic version (ECV) at the end of pregnancy.

Before the mid-1970s, ECV was usually attempted before term because of the belief that the procedure would seldom be successful at term. Subsequent studies showed that, with the use of tocolysis, ECV could be achieved in a substantial proportion of women with breech presentation at term. ECV at term differs in many fundamental ways from that performed before term. These include the fact that the fetus is mature and may be delivered more readily in the event of complications. This study shows that ECV at term is associated with a significant reduction in non-cephalic births and caesarean section. There is no significant effect on perinatal mortality. The Cochrane Database disc includes an excellent video in which Professor Justus Hofmeyr gently, firmly, with skilled hands and great sensitivity, coaxes a baby round from breech to cephalic.

A study in South Africa reveals that many younger obstetricians do not do ECV, do not know how to do it, or think it is not worth the bother. By 1993 the UK caesarean section rate for breech deliveries was 69%. It is likely to be a good deal higher than that now. Yet six randomised controlled trials have revealed that two out of three babies can be turned, and will stay vertex for birth if ECV is performed after 37 weeks, or even early in labour. In fact, ECV halves the caesarean section rates for breech-presenting babies. The Royal College of Obstetricians and Gynaecologists has recommended that 'all women at term with an uncomplicated pregnancy and breech presentation should be offered ECV'.[27] In a major London hospital the caesarean rate in women with breech babies in the first 9 months of 1997 was 90%.

Even if the baby cannot be turned, vaginal birth may be a sensible option. A lot depends on the skills and experience of the obstetrician or midwife. There has been only one randomised controlled trial comparing breech vaginal birth with caesarean delivery. As a result of the findings of this study, all over the world women are now told that it is dangerous to attempt a vaginal birth and the only safe method of delivery is by caesarean.

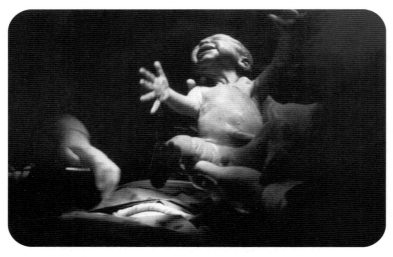

Although sometimes the best option for the mother, a caesarean can be a shock for the baby

This trial has been criticised on the grounds that it was methodologically flawed. Many of the 121 centres that participated in the trial were in North America, and some tripled their vaginal delivery rate overnight when they entered the trial, since they were instructed that if their breech vaginal delivery rate was less than 40% they must either withdraw from the research or increase the rate. They may not have had the special skills and experience to do vaginal breech births. In effect, they had to fling caution to the winds and up the rate 'beyond their previous comfort level'. That 'comfort level' is important for safety.

Another problem with this trial was that all women with breech babies were assigned a similar risk status, whereas clearly some vaginal births are trickier than others. A woman who has already given birth vaginally, who is at 38 weeks with a 3000 g baby in a frank breech presentation with the head well flexed, and when labour is advancing well, is low risk. In effect, the research 'homogenised both the study population and clinical intervention, resulted in an average level of care in an average population, limiting the trial's reliability in countries showing above average skill and in women of below average risk'.

It used to be claimed that 'once a caesarean, always a caesarean'. But this is ridiculous. Many women who have had previous caesareans are able to deliver another baby vaginally. Two obstetricians at the University of Toronto undertook a Medline database search on all articles published in English in the journals, including meta-analyses and retrospective and prospective studies, to determine antenatal factors that may predict successful vaginal births after caesarean (VBAC). Even women who had previous cephalopelvic disproportion had a 75% chance of giving birth vaginally. The more caesareans a woman had previously undergone, the lower her chance of success. A previous vaginal birth was a very good prognostic indication of being able to give birth vaginally, especially if the vaginal birth followed a caesarean. Even big babies did not make a caesarean inevitable. More than half the women with big babies were able to have vaginal births, and uterine rupture was not increased. More than two-thirds of women with post-dates pregnancies had vaginal births too. The authors concluded that 'there are few absolute contraindications to attempted VBAC' and that most will be successful.[28] Research in Scotland reveals that women who have undergone an instrumental vaginal birth who go on to have another pregnancy opt for vaginal birth, even though they are afraid of what the experience will be like, rather than a caesarean next time round. In this study, 94% of the women achieved vaginal birth after a previous caesarean.[29]

I run a Birth Crisis Network to enable women who have had distressing births to talk about them with other women who understand, listen reflectively and enable the woman gradually to come to terms with the experience of having been disempowered during a major life event. Many of these women express gratitude to their obstetricians immediately after an emergency caesarean or other operative procedure, but become distressed a couple of months later. They feel cheated, lose self-esteem, and suffer flashbacks and panic attacks. Post-traumatic stress disorder after childbirth is only just now being recognised by obstetricians. General practitioners are coming to realise, albeit slowly, that women who are distressed after childbirth do not necessarily suffer from postnatal depression and should not be treated with antidepressants or tranquillisers. They need to talk. They need someone to *listen*.

Every week I hear accounts of horrendous experiences of obstetric management. Women's bodies are treated like machines that are always in danger of crashing. Women describe being made to lie on their back for hours, harpooned to electronic machines, intravenous drips and catheters, before ending up with an emergency caesarean section. It is understandable that women who have been through an experience like that prefer, with their next baby, to have an elective caesarean under controlled conditions, with guaranteed pain relief. For many modern women obstetric management has made the birth room a torture chamber, and elective caesarean section offers release from it. Vaginal birth, and its consequences of a damaged perineum, pelvic floor, bladder and bowels, has become such a traumatic experience that they can only face having another baby if it is by elective caesarean section. These women are not 'too posh to push'. They are survivors of torture. Their choice is carefully considered and rational. Planned surgery is likely to be more comfortable than high-tech managed labour with cumulative interventions in a hostile and inhumane environment that inhibits their spontaneous behaviour and impedes normal labour. We should be challenging not only the high caesarean rate, but also the aggressive management of vaginal birth and the many ways in which physiological processes are disturbed.

Persuasion and manipulation

It is not only women who have already been traumatised by a distressing birth who opt for a caesarean. Most women, if told by an obstetrician that a caesarean is best for the baby, go along with professional advice. Obstetricians increasingly advise instrumental or caesarean delivery as a quick-fix solution to *potential* problems, as well as those actually confronted. Elina Hemminki concludes her commentary on the study of obstetricians' attitudes by saying: 'An intriguing question is what has created this favourable attitude of London obstetricians toward caesarean sections, a view in contradiction with scientific literature. If obstetricians have opinions that lack scientific basis, informed choice by a patient is impossible'.[30]

In a discourse analysis of discussion between members of an obstetric team in a large regional maternity unit in which they were recorded in their everyday interactions with colleagues, Julia Simpson shows how pregnant women are categorised. Here the consultant is talking:

> *One of the problems is that women generally tend to be very self-centred and selfish but they don't always get the chance to express that or to rectify the situation. But when they are pregnant then somebody has to listen to them* [registrar laughs]. *They are the centre of attention. The whole obstetric world*

is set up to focus on the pregnant woman and they are going to take advantage of it. They come along here and they ask questions 'Oh where does the Venflon go?' and 'How long will I be in the operating theatre?' I don't think they are really interested at all, it's just that they want to continue to be the centre of attention and the focus of the whole show.[31]

Women are also perceived as manipulative. The registrar says:

I think that as obstetricians what we need to learn is to start being very manipulative with the women, because they are being very manipulative with us. Our only defence is going to be manipulative back because our normal standard approach which is using logical, factual information and sense isn't working. It's not going to work. That approach is not going to work.[32]

Julia Simpson states that the obstetrician places himself in the role of victim:

The undisclosed 'hidden agenda' in these circumstances is that it is not the pregnant woman who is at risk; it is the senior team members who perceive that they are at risk. As obstetricians they risk losing their control of the practitioner/client encounter and therefore their ability to maintain their professional authority when negotiating treatment options.[33]

The registrar describes his interaction with the pregnant women as 'a battle' – 'It's like a battle between you, that you know that you are going to win'. Julia Simpson concludes: 'The language of resistance and defence permeates the talk about their clients and they arrive at the conclusion that pregnant women want to blame and "trap" the professional'.

This discourse analysis illustrates how the members of an obstetric team use 'the rhetoric of risk ... to construct, assemble and magnify a professional definition of risk in circumstances where none may actually exist for the obstetric client. Even if there are no obstetric problems at all with a woman's pregnancy, the rhetoric of risk is being used to construct birth as a situation of inherent risk requiring expert technical management by obstetricians'. In this way the woman is manipulated into agreeing to, or better still, choosing, an elective caesarean section.[34]

Women seek caesareans not just because they cannot face pain, or because they want to keep their vaginas 'honeymoon fresh', but because they hope they can maintain some control over what is done to them, and because they are told that caesareans are safer for the baby. They are warned about the risk of cerebral palsy, for example. However, whereas caesarean rates have gone up by leaps and bounds over the last 30 years, rates of cerebral palsy have stayed the same. Women are rarely told that the risks to the mother are higher with caesarean than vaginal birth. That includes the risk of dying, as well as pelvic infections, harmful side-effects of anaesthesia, operative injury, haemorrhage, uterine rupture, and the psychological consequences of surgery.[35]

Women are also not told that one of the best ways of avoiding a caesarean is to have a woman companion with them in labour, as well as, or instead of, a partner. Although the Dublin method of active management was introduced with the hope of cutting the rise in caesarean sections, it has failed to achieve this. Ten randomised controlled trials have shown that the constant presence of a birth companion is more effective in checking the rise in caesarean sections.[36] I, for one, am certain that human companionship is more humane.

Do most women really want a caesarean?

Statements about caesareans being a 'woman's choice' ignore the power differential between women and obstetricians. By reinforcing the idea that caesareans are completely safe, easy, efficient and desirable for the baby's well-being – and even its life – and claiming that with a caesarean a woman avoids pain and injury, an emergency procedure has become routine practice. The medical system has co-opted the notion of choice.

References

1. Al-Muftir R, McCarthy A, Fisk NM 1996 Obstetricians' personal choice and mode of delivery. Lancet 347(9000):544

2. Gabbe SG, Holzman GB 2001 Obstetricians' choice of delivery [letter]. Lancet 357(9257):722

3. Francis WJA 1960 Disturbances of bladder function in relation to pregnancy. Journal of Obstetrics and Gynaecology of the British Empire 67:353–366

4. Francis WJA 1960 The onset of stress incontinence. Journal of Obstetrics and Gynaecology of the British Empire 67:899–903

5. Brown A 1997 Medical ethics – respecting patient choice. Paper presented at The Royal Society of Medicine, London

6. Are too many made to give birth this way? No says Dickinson Cowan, Yes says Sheila Kitzinger. The Express, 19 February 1997

7. Nielsen TF, Otterblad Olausson P, Ingemarsson I 1994 The cesarean section rate in Sweden: the end of the rise. Birth 21(1):34–38

8. Thomas J, Paranjothy S 2001 Royal College of Obstetricians and Gynaecologists Clinical Effectiveness Support Unit. National sentinel caesarean section audit report. London: RCOG Press. Available at: http://www.rcog.org.uk/resources/public/nscs_audit.pdf (accessed November 2004)

9. Leyshon L 2004 Integrating caseloads across a whole service: the Torbay model. MIDIRS Midwifery Digest 14(1):59–61

10. Thomas J, Paranjothy S 2001 The national sentinel caesarean section audit report. London: Royal College of Obstetricians and Gynaecologists

11. Mohajer M 2004 The hub and spoke model of care. MIDIRS Midwifery Digest 14(1):518–519

12. Gomes UA, Silva AAM, Bettiol H, et al 1999 Risk factors for the increasing caesarean section rate in southeast Brazil: a comparison of two birth stories, 1978–1979, 1994. International Journal of Epidemiology 28:687–694

13. Pai M 2000 Caesarean section controversy: a debate is needed on caesarean section rates in India [letter]. BMJ 320(7241):1072

14. Dumont A, de Bernis L, Bouvier-Colle MH, et al 2001 Caesarean section rate for maternal indication in sub-Saharan Africa: a systematic review. Lancet 358(9290):1328–1333

15. Potter JE, Berquó E, Perpétuo IH, et al 2001 Unwanted caesarean sections among public and private patients in Brazil: prospective study. BMJ 323(7322):1155–1158

16. Behague DP, Victora CG, Barros FC 2002 Consumer demand for caesarean sections in Brazil: informed study linking ethnographic and epidemiological methods. BMJ 324(7343):942–945

17. Hopkins K 2000 Are Brazilian women really choosing to deliver by caesarean? Society of Scientific Medicine 51:725–740

18. Bettiol H, Barbieri MA, da Silva AA, et al 2002 Consumer demand for caesarean sections in Brazil. Demand is affected by mothers' perception of good health care [letter]. BMJ 325(7359):335

19. Potter JE, Hopkins K 2002 Consumer demand for caesarean sections in Brazil. Demand should be assessed rather than inferred. BMJ 325(7359):335–336

20. Murray SF 2000 Relation between private health insurance and high rates of caesarean section in Chile: qualitative and quantitative study. BMJ 321(7275):1501–1505

21. Ventura SJ, Martin JA, Curtin SC, et al 1997 Report of final natality statistics, 1995. Monthly Vital Statistics Report 45(11 Suppl):13

22. Enkin M, Keirse MJNC, Neilson J, et al 2000 Guide to effective care in pregnancy and childbirth, 3rd edn. Oxford: Oxford University Press, pp 270–275

23. Haverkamp AD, Orleans M, Langendoerfer S, et al 1979 A controlled trial of the differential effects of intrapartum fetal monitoring. American Journal of Obstetrics and Gynacology 134(4):399–412

24. Bassindale C 1997 Caesarean section. Frank 212–214

25. Lieberman E, Cohen A, Lang JM, et al 1995 The association of epidural anesthesia with cesarean section in low risk women. American Journal of Obstetrics and Gynecology 172(1):276

26. Murphy DJ, Fowlie PW, McGuire W 2004 Obstetric issues in preterm birth. BMJ 329(7469):783–786

27. Royal College of Obstetricians and Gynaecologists 1993 Effective procedures in obstetrics suitable for audit. Manchester: Royal College of Obstetricians and Gynaecologists Medical Audit Unit, p 2

28. Brill Y, Windrim R 2003 Vaginal birth after caesarean section: review of antenatal predictors of success. Journal of Obstetrics and Gynaecology of Canada 25(4):275–286

29. Bahl R, Strachan B, Murphy DJ 2004 Outcome of subsequent pregnancy three years after previous operative delivery in the second stage of labour [short study]. BMJ 328:311–313

30. Hemminki E 1997 Cesarean sections: women's choice for giving birth? Birth 24(2):124–125

31. Simpson J 2004 Negotiating elective cesarean section: an obstetric team perspective. In: Kirkham M (ed) Informed choice in maternity care. New York: Palgrave MacMillan, p 224

32. Simpson J 2004 Negotiating elective cesarean section: an obstetric team perspective. In: Kirkham M (ed) Informed choice in maternity care. New York: Palgrave MacMillan, p 228

33. Simpson J 2004 Negotiating elective cesarean section: an obstetric team perspective. In: Kirkham M (ed) Informed choice in maternity care. New York: Palgrave MacMillan, p 230

34. Simpson J 2004 Negotiating elective cesarean section: an obstetric team perspective. In: Kirkham M (ed) Informed choice in maternity care. New York: Palgrave MacMillan, pp 231–232

35. Enkin MW, Keirse MJNC, Renfrew MJ, et al 1995 Pregnancy and childbirth module. Cochrane database of systematic reviews. London: BMJ Publishing Group

36. Hodnett ED 1995 Support from caregivers during childbirth. In: Enkin MW, Keirse MJNC, Renfrew MJ, Neilson JP (eds) Pregnancy and childbirth module. Cochrane database of systematic reviews. London: BMJ Publishing Group

10
Court-ordered caesareans

The legality of compulsory section after a fetus has been made a ward of court is being fought in the USA state by state. The basic issue is whether the rights of the fetus override the rights of a mother. Lynn Paltrow, Executive Director of National Advocates for Pregnant Women, who represent women charged with child abuse because they suffer drug addiction during pregnancy, says: 'Even if you think of the fetus as a person, in America we don't allow the courts to decide between two people and order one to undergo surgery for the other'.[1] Colleen Connell, a lawyer with the American Civil Liberties Union, explains, 'It's a well-established common law that an adult has the right to make medical decisions on their own behalf. Pregnancy does not strip a woman of that legal right'. Describing a case in which she represented a woman who won her case against a hospital that was seeking to force her to have a caesarean section, she said: 'The Illinois court ruled a woman's right to make medical decisions on her own behalf does not evaporate just because she's pregnant. To do anything else would make a woman hostage to the fetus from the moment of conception to the moment of birth'.[2]

I was lecturing in Turin just after the judgement by three Law Lords in Britain that a court-ordered caesarean on a woman in her right mind was illegal. The Italian midwives were astonished. They told me that women in Italy are often overruled in the best interests of the baby, and since obstetricians are the experts, their decision is authoritative and sacrosanct. They believed that no one would question a decision made by an Italian obstetrician against a woman's wishes. When I discussed this with one of the midwives she commented: 'We have priests and doctors. They are very powerful and women in childbirth are terribly vulnerable'.

In Britain, the law is unequivocal: compulsory surgical or invasive treatment of a male or female patient is illegal. It is as illegal to force a woman to submit to caesarean section as it would be to force anyone to give bone marrow or a kidney, even to someone who desperately needed a transplant, and even if that person was his own child. It is an issue of human rights.

A 30-year-old veterinary nurse registered with a London general practitioner when she was 36 weeks pregnant and asked for a home birth.[3] The doctor examined her and told her that she had pre-eclampsia and must come into hospital immediately for induction. She declined, saying that she wanted a natural birth and would go to Wales and have her baby in a cave there, rather than go into hospital. The doctor called in a social worker who tried to convince her that she should be admitted to St. George's Hospital, Tooting, for induction. The mother was crying. She said the baby's father had left her. When it was suggested that she was depressed, she admitted that she probably was. She was subjected to cross-questioning for hours on end until late into the night. Her blood pressure (not surprisingly) remained high. A psychiatrist was called in and the social worker made an application under section 2 of the 1983 Mental Health Act and arranged for her to be forcibly admitted to a mental hospital and detained for 'assessment'.

The mother three times refused her consent, recorded in writing her 'extreme objection to *any* medical or surgical intervention' and made it 'absolutely clear that it [a caesarean section] is against my wishes and I should consider it an assault upon my person'. She wrote, 'I have always held very strong views with regard to medical and surgical treatments for myself, and particularly wish to allow nature to "take its course", without intervention. I fully understand that in certain circumstances this may endanger my life. I see death as a natural and inevitable end-point to certain conditions, and that natural events should not be interfered with. It is not a belief attached to the fact of my being pregnant, and would apply equally to any condition arising'. She called a firm of solicitors, talked to a lawyer for half-an-hour, and said she would seek legal advice first thing in the morning.

But that was not to be. Just before midnight she was transported to a maternity hospital. An application was made to a judge in a Family Court, in an emergency hearing, who was told by the hospital authorities that she had been in labour for 24 hours and that this was a life or death situation with only minutes to spare. In fact, she was not in labour. Although her psychiatrist considered that her 'capacity for consent was intact', the court was not told of this. The judge was not notified that 'Ms S' had already instructed solicitors, and the hearing was even kept secret from the woman herself. The judge failed to ask whether she was mentally competent and ruled that she could be compelled to have a caesarean – as if it were a treatment for mental illness. The caesarean was performed. Ms S offered no physical resistance, but said that she was submitting to surgery against her will.

After the caesarean, and following a restless night, Ms S said that she was very angry that the hospital had gone against her wishes, and complained of physical assault. She at first rejected her baby. Five days later she was returned to the mental hospital, where she was examined by a psychiatrist who said that there were 'no current abnormalities in her mental state'. She was released from detention and immediately discharged herself.

She sued the hospital. In this important case three judges ruled that both the detention and the caesarean operation were unlawful, even though a High Court judge had sanctioned it. The woman had a right to damages against the National Health Service for false imprisonment and trespass to her person. They also ruled that any declaration made in a court hearing when the patient is not represented does not protect doctors and hospitals from being sued for trespass. The court reaffirmed the right of any competent adult, male or female, to refuse medical or surgical intervention, even if the result was certain death for the individual or for a fetus.

The Mental Health Act cannot be used to detain an individual against her will merely if her thinking process is unusual, even bizarre and irrational, and contrary to the views of the majority of the community. That is a fundamental constitutional principle, which can be traced back to the Magna Carta of 1297.

The judges laid down guidelines 'to avoid any recurrence of the unsatisfactory events recorded in this judgement'. Doctors and hospital managers must consider, as a priority, whether a patient is mentally competent. If so, the individual's decision has to be respected. If there is a court hearing, the patient should be allowed to consult a solicitor, and must be represented at the hearing.

The British Medical Association welcomed the ruling. A spokeswoman said that 'the fact that a woman has moral obligations to her baby, does not mean the health professionals or the courts can compel her to fulfil them'.[4]

When an obstetrician assumes responsibility in this way, giving prime consideration to the fetus as a patient and seeing the woman merely as a container for it, she is reduced to being a non-person. Not only was there a clear presumption of maternal incompetence and refusal to consider the woman's views and feelings in this case, but also poor communication and documentation and blatant deception. Although health professionals may have strong views about the need for a specific treatment, a line must always been drawn between advice and coercion.

References

1. Paltrow L 2004 Speaking on national public radio, USA, 17 January 2004
2. Connell C 2004 Speaking on national public radio, USA, 17 January 2004
3. Draft Judgement in Supreme Court of Judicature Court of Appeal, UK, before Lady Justice Butler-Sloss, Lord Justice Judge and Lord Justice Robert Walker, 7 May 1998
4. Dyer C 1998 Trusts face damages after forcing women to have caesareans. BMJ 316(7143):1480

11
Birth plans

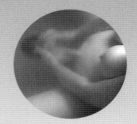

Why not draw up a birth plan? [a partogram] Why not reduce the patient's anxiety by telling her how we expect her labour to progress and when she may deliver? After all, none of us likes to go to the airport not knowing when our plane is going to take off or land.[1]

That is one obstetrician's idea of a birth plan – a system of active management imposed on a woman whether she likes it or not. There are other obstetricians who see a birth plan as a shopping list in which a patient makes demands about care, and thus as a sign that the patient is going to be 'difficult'. They say birth plans are unrealistic, uncompromising, confrontational and anxiety arousing. It is true that some are like this. Yet, in one sense, a hospital gets the birth plans it deserves. In any hospital where it is known that there are routine interventions in birth, those women who dare make a birth plan tend to concentrate on interventions they wish to avoid: 'No induction of labour. No drugs of any kind. No episiotomy. Baby to have nothing but breast milk'. Such plans can be a reaction to real, not imagined, threats.

In spite of this, birth plans have become part of the birth scene, even if accepted grudgingly and readily dismissed in practice, in both North America and the UK. Within any birth culture, subjects that are *not* argued about are as interesting as those which are constantly being debated. In the 1980s and 1990s, birth plans were the topic of often heated discussion. This is no longer the case.

Although some obstetricians still tend to reject women's self-created birth plans, and may go so far as to treat them as evidence of mental instability, it should be remembered that in the UK around 70% of births are conducted by midwives. So the midwife's attitude to a woman's birth plan is vital. Already in 1986, when senior midwives in England and Wales replied to a questionnaire sent by Dr Jo Garcia of the National Perinatal Epidemiology Unit (NPEU), it emerged that 33% of hospitals encouraged birth plans as a matter of policy.[2, 3] Now midwives incorporate birth plans into care. Many are at ease with them, and use the discussion that results as an educational opportunity for getting to know each woman and understanding her needs.

This is not 'alternative' but mainstream care. One National Health Service (NHS) hospital, for example, has a system by which all women are visited at home by a midwife in the third trimester to discuss the conduct of labour and delivery.[4] The midwife offers a ready-made birth plan form that lists each common procedure, asks the woman to indicate whether she would like it, wants to avoid it, or has no strong views, and inquires if she has any other special wishes. This is kept with the woman's records, and on admission to hospital the midwife on duty studies the plan so that care can be tailored to that woman's preferences and priorities.

When, after exploring the idea with Penny Simkin in Seattle,[5] I first suggested the use of birth plans in the UK, I did not realise how quickly they would catch on with mothers and midwives, even though they often turned out to be different from what I was proposing. One thing we have learned is that when a birth plan is not part of ongoing antenatal education, so that each woman has the information necessary to weigh up the pros and cons of different practices, it may become a matter of superficial, casual, even instant choice – rather like choosing between cans of beans in a supermarket display. It does nothing to enable her to be more in control of what is happening.

In one hospital, for example, where midwives are opposed to routine episiotomies, some women requested episiotomy in their birth plan because they believed that if they did not have one they would be bound to tear in an uncontrolled way. The midwives were nonplussed. When the time came, however, and the midwife had formed a relationship with the woman in labour, 'reassurance at the time of delivery proved sufficient and no episiotomies were performed unless there was an indication'.[4]

Printed birth plans

Another risk with birth plans is that the medical system appropriates them as a symbol of consumerism in order to assert the power of an institution. Observing that women were starting to write down what they wanted, during the 1980s hospitals started to devise their own printed forms, on which women had only to tick boxes or underline 'Yes' or 'No'. I did a content analysis of responses to the NPEU questionnaire from the 47 hospitals which said they encouraged birth plans and submitted documentation about them. Many were using them to reassure pregnant women and to achieve patient compliance. These strategies can be categorised under the following six headings.

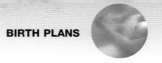

Framing

Boundaries are drawn around a limited range of options. Many of these choices are trivial. A woman may be invited to decide whether she wishes to wear a hospital gown or her own 'nightie', or whether or not she would like to have a bath after delivery. Options may also be presented as personal choices which are, in fact, part of standard hospital practice – for example, 'Would you like to hold your baby after delivery?' This question only makes sense if a woman is asked if she wants to hold her baby immediately at birth or if she prefers the baby to be washed first. It then becomes an acknowledgement of cultural differences.

Shrinkage

The woman is invited to make a free choice, but little space is provided on the printed form in which to record her wishes. When birth plans consist merely of a series of 'Yes' or 'No' tick boxes, or unequivocal statements 'I agree to this' or 'I refuse permission for that', it can put a midwife in an intolerable position. Instead of having a relationship with the woman in childbirth, she is like a supermarket check-out clerk, recording preselected sales goods, and unable to use her professional skills to support a woman through the birth experience. It is no wonder that midwives have resisted birth plans of that kind.[6]

Marginalisation

In this case the wording of the plan indicates that certain preferences are abnormal. Any woman who does not do what 'most' women choose is at risk of being singled out as 'an anxious patient'. One birth plan form, for example, stated: 'Fetal monitoring by electronic machine is welcomed by the majority of mothers – any fears or questions?'

Therapising

When birth plans are seen primarily as a means of 'reassuring' the patient, there may also be, as in the last example, an attempt to get mothers to disclose their fears and anxieties. Responses to birth plans are interpreted as a symptom of pathology requiring treatment or, at least, firm handling.

The foregone conclusion

Options are often presented in such a way as to pre-judge the issue. In one leaflet women were asked whether they wished to 'correct a slow labour' by an intravenous drip. No further information was offered about why a labour might be slow or why it needed correcting, or any alternative ways in which it might be 'corrected'. Women were also asked whether they wished to have an injection to 'prevent bleeding' in the third stage; again, without any explanation or discussion. Women cannot make informed choices unless they know the side-effects of interventions and alternative ways of dealing with any deviations from the normal.

Emotional blackmail

Women are told that their babies are in danger if they do not obey. One form required a woman's consent 'to agree to guidance from the doctor or midwife for the safety of herself or the baby' and announced: 'The procedures we recommend to you are tried and tested to make childbirth as safe as possible for mother and baby'. So, it was implied, do not question the experts.

Asserting medical control over women

At its most basic level, in any hospital where care is fragmented, as it is in most maternity units, the birth plan provides a nucleus around which some continuity can be achieved. Midwives agree, however, that birth plans work best when their creation helps to focus the relationship between a woman and her caregivers. If contingency plans are also constructed, they enable midwives and doctors to understand a woman's priorities when there are deviations from the normal.

Few birth plan documents designed by caregivers ask the woman whether she would like to give birth at home or in hospital. Even when this choice is

Dear Tessa.

I have made you an appointment to see me at my midwives clinic at the Nuffield Health Centre on

.... Mon. 26ᶠ July. 2.00 pm ....

This appointment is for me to make the necessary booking arrangements for you to have your baby at the John Radcliffe Hospital.

If the time and date is not convenient for you, please would you phone the receptionist and she will change it for you.

Yours sincerely,

Midwife.

I gather too Dr Maxwell that you would like to discuss a home water birth.

The original letter to pregnant women assumed that birth would be in hospital

available the result may be a mixture of marginalisation and emotional blackmail. One leaflet for patients, *Home or Hospital Birth?*, started off by stating: 'Any woman who becomes pregnant has increased the risk to her life. Every couple who decide to start a family has decided that it is worth taking a small risk with the mother's life for the sake of having children'. It went on to discuss the 'known risks of a home birth': 'If the baby does not start to breathe properly after the birth, it is impossible to provide the same apparatus or expert help that is immediately available in a hospital. Death or permanent handicap could sometimes happen because of this ... Because experienced midwives and doctors have all had experience of the problems which can happen unexpectedly and very suddenly in childbirth, they almost all recommend that in Britain today it is advisable for all births to take place in hospital'. Dealing with a 'Previous Bad Hospital Experience', the leaflet states, 'Fortunately, these days in most hospitals, this kind of experience is being reported less and less' (no evidence is presented for this statement) 'and the best and safest response, especially for any birth which has not been assessed as "low risk" is not to have a home birth, but rather to build up a relationship of trust and mutual respect with the hospital team'. There was a form to be signed by the consultant obstetrician stressing the view that hospital birth is medically safer and that 'although I always personally recommend hospital birth (if only to reduce the severe stress inevitably caused to your Family Doctor and Midwife), I can also appreciate your willingness to accept a possibly increased medical risk for the sake of other possible advantages'. A risk rating was assigned to the patient, ranging through very low/low/significantly high/seriously high/dangerous. A useful research project at this hospital might have been a psychological study to measure the anxiety of patients who were presented with this document compared with that of those who had not been shown it.

The reason often given for constructing hospital birth plan leaflets is that they improve communication and it is expected that this will result in more 'informed consent'. But an equally valid outcome is *informed refusal*. Informed consent echoes through the new 'birth speak'. As we have seen in Chapter 7, refusal is rarely mentioned, and may be perceived as a failure in patient management.

Birth plans employed in this way give little or no opportunity for women to explore the issues involved and decide on their own priorities. Rather than being educational tools that help midwives to understand women's needs more accurately, the birth plans are used to achieve patient compliance.

The birth culture

A group of midwives revealed that birth plans were still a source of irritation to some midwives in the late 1990s.[7] This investigation tells us more about those who did the research than about the women in their care. The authors stated: 'Midwifery is unique and a speciality in that patients may *dictate* their management'. 'Birth plans may *put pressure on midwives* to comply with patients' requests. Some birth plans may appear to be *unreasonable*. It is not surprising that their study revealed that 'Birth plans may adversely affect the outcome of labour'. Women who made birth plans had more forceps and ventouse deliveries, more caesareans, and more interventions of all kinds. They attributed this to the existence of the birth plan, rather than investigating the responses of members of staff to women who offered birth plans, trying to find out whether there was a poor relationship between them and their clients and, if so, how this might be improved. It was a frightening thought that any woman who produced a birth plan was likely to end up with an operative delivery because preparing such a plan had 'provoked some degree of annoyance' in the professionals caring for her.

A significant omission from the study was any mention of child-bearing women's own experiences of birth plans. The research should have included discussion with women, antenatally and after birth, concerning their views of how birth plans are used, with suggestions from them about how plans might be employed more effectively. It is when a woman doubts whether anyone is listening to what she is saying that she may produce a birth plan that seems 'unreasonable'. When birth plans are not used as a matter of course, part of the normal dialogue between caregivers and women, they are often an expression of a woman's anxiety that her labour will be managed in an authoritarian way. This may be a realistic fear.

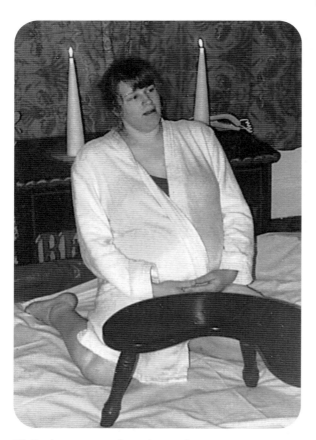

Research in Australia to assess how birth plans were used in Victoria revealed that women who constructed birth plans were more likely to be satisfied with

Birth plans are not just about what a woman does *not* want. A mother in early labour creates a space with strong spiritual focus

pain relief and significantly less likely to have an operative vaginal delivery, but were no more satisfied with the care they received than were women who did not make a plan and were not especially involved in making decisions about care. The authors called for a randomised trial to gather further evidence. However, two-thirds of birth-plan mothers thought there were definite advantages in writing down their preferences ahead of time.[8]

Another Australian study[9] showed that birth plans empower women by increasing their knowledge and understanding of birth practices and helping them make enormous choices, and demonstrated the commitment of caregivers to recognising and supporting diversity. It built a 'therapeutic alliance' between client and caregiver. But even in this study, in two Sydney hospitals where 90% of women used birth plans, one-third did not feel they were encouraged to ask questions. The authors attribute this to the power imbalance between clients and professionals, lack of time, language and cultural barriers, and 'embarrassment about appearing ignorant and uninformed'. Yet, in the long run, not having enough time to discuss your wishes fully, being unable to communicate easily, and being anxious about appearing ignorant are all symptoms of a power imbalance. This is the heart of the matter.

Mothers and midwives

Some midwives are skilled at using the rhetoric of choice while persuading women to make what they see as the correct choices. In a study of how Informed Choice leaflets were used in practice, Mavis Kirkham and Helen Stapleton found that midwives talked about 'woman-centred care' and 'facilitating informed choice' 'whilst their clinical behaviour was routinised and rule governed'.[10]

In consultant units most midwives spoke of 'informed choice' but actually concentrated on 'checking'. 'Experience of a culture of powerlessness left midwives ill-equipped to empower their clients, as they lacked the confidence or sense of their own power that is needed before power can be shared'.[11] The conclusion is that 'most of the midwives observed nurtured the maternity service and their employing organisation. They acted as the shock absorbers which took the stress within that service and made its routinised system able to continue'.[12] Under such circumstances talk about birth plans is employed to lead women into thinking that they have genuine choice, when they may have none.

The creation of a birth plan has the potential to be an educational process for all concerned. It can help midwives, as well as mothers. It triggers an active search for information that is evidence-based. It stimulates dialogue between the woman and her caregivers and prepares the way for a partnership in which the caregivers understand the woman's priorities and preferences. A birth plan can be one expression of a good working relationship between the two parties. Moreover, they are *equal* partners, bringing their own skills and knowledge, recognising those which the other person has, and knowing their limits. The birth plan also brings into the open exactly what a woman expects of her birth companions and helps them talk together about the kind of support she wants during childbirth.

Birth plans have been criticised for being based on the false assumption that women are not able to make decisions when they are in labour because they are not considered mentally competent. A birth plan fills the gap where their brains should be. In a paper about this, Heather Cahill asserts that 'Encouraging women to complete birth plans simply reinforces the assumption of incompetence. The implicit message is that, while women may be indeed competent at the time they complete the plan, at the onset of labour and delivery they will no longer be so' because they are in such an anxious state and in so much pain that they cannot make a rational decision.[13] This is an interesting theory, but we can accept that labour is usually an overwhelming experience without believing that therefore women are out of their minds. In the spaces between contractions, they often have sharp mental clarity.

We all know how birth plans are misused – the ones that are mere shopping lists, for example, and that do not allow any flexibility. They are often perceived as binding contracts, thus putting pressure on a woman to stick to her plan come hell or high water. She must be able to change her mind at any time, and to do so without persuasion. If, because she has made a birth plan, she is not allowed to change her mind, far from being empowering, the plan disempowers her. A birth plan must never be used as a quick and easy short-term solution to poor continuity of care and a substitute for good communication.

It is important that every birth plan should include contingency plans in case a birth is not straightforward. It is not that different from a plan for a cycling or walking trip. What if it rains? What if the going is too tough? It should be possible to modify the plan depending on how the woman feels at the time. She needs to think ahead and to discuss what she would wish to happen if her labour proved to be slow and tiring, for example, or if pain cannot be handled in the ways that she hoped. This can be a constructive, practical discussion in which alternatives are explored.

A vital element of a birth plan is that it should be part of a continuing relationship during the pregnancy between a woman and her caregivers, and one in which there is growing understanding. Thus it entails continuity of care and, best of all, continuity of carer. It takes time. The creation of a birth plan is a *process*.

I have a friend, a strong advocate of the birth plan, who experienced a fetal death at 33 weeks. She told me that she decided, under the circumstances, on an epidural, asked that she and her husband could hold the baby immediately, and arranged to cuddle the baby in bed right through the night before saying goodbye to him in the morning. Although her labour was very different from what she expected, she was able to state with clarity the human values and beliefs that were important to her in this major life event. That is what birth plans are all about.

References

1. Borges S 1991 The importance of artificial rupture of membranes in early labour as part of active management of labour. Obstetrics and Gynaecology Product News 19–20

2. Garcia J, Garforth S, Ayers S 1987 The policy and practice in midwifery study: introduction and methods. Midwifery 3(1):2–9

3. Garcia J, Garforth S 1991 Midwifery policies and policy making. In: Robinson S, Thomson AM (eds) Midwives, research and childbirth, vol II. London: Chapman & Hall

4. Ekeocha CEO, Jackson P 1985 The 'birth plan' experience. British Journal of Obstetrics and Gynaecology 92:97–101

5. Simkin P, Reinke C 1980 Planning your baby's birth. Seattle, WA: Pennypress

6. Kitzinger S 1987 Freedom and choice in childbirth. London: Penguin Books (Published in the USA as: Your baby, your way: making pregnancy decisions and birth plans. New York: Pantheon Books, 1987)

7. Jones MH, Barik S, Mangune HH, et al 1998 Do birth plans adversely affect the outcome of labour? British Journal of Midwifery 6(1):38–41

8. Brown SJ, Lumley J 1998 Communication and decision-making in labour: do birth plans make a difference? Health Expectations 1998; 1(2):106–116

9. Moore M, Hopper U 1995 Do birth plans empower women? Evaluation of a hospital birth plan. Birth 22(1):29–36

10. Kirkham M, Stapleton H 2004 The culture of the maternity services in Wales and England as a barrier to informed choice. In: Kirkham M (ed) Informed choice in maternity care. New York: Palgrave Macmillan, p 131

11. Kirkham M, Stapleton H 2004 The culture of the maternity services in Wales and England as a barrier to informed choice. In: Kirkham M (ed) Informed choice in maternity care. New York: Palgrave Macmillan, p 142

12. Kirkham M, Stapleton H 2004 The culture of the maternity services in Wales and England as a barrier to informed choice. In: Kirkham M (ed) Informed choice in maternity care. New York: Palgrave Macmillan, p 143

13. Cahill H 1999 An Orwellian scenario: court ordered caesarean section and women's autonomy. Nursing Ethics 6(6):494–505

12
Home birth

Many of us working in the childbirth movement felt for years that we were beating our heads against the brick wall of a rigid medical system that treated women merely as containers for the fetus. Yet occasionally we have become aware of the fruits of our efforts and realise that after all we are making progress. This is what happened when we opened the House of Commons' *Report on Maternity Services*[1] (the Winterton Report) in 1992, and saw startling proposals for change toward woman-centred care. Right at the beginning it stated: 'There is no convincing and compelling evidence that hospitals give a better guarantee of safety for the majority of mothers and babies', and its first conclusion was unequivocal: 'The policy of encouraging all women to give birth in hospitals cannot be justified on grounds of safety'.

This all-party Health Committee examined carefully evidence not only from research and professional bodies but also from women's and consumer organisations. The result was that it challenged what it called the 'unproven assumption' that hospital, by definition, provided optimal care for mothers and babies. In fact it stated that 'the experience of the hospital environment too often deters women from asserting control over their own bodies and too often leaves them feeling that, in retrospect, they have not had the best labour and delivery they could have hoped for'. It acknowledged that women want choice as to the place of birth, fragmented care is dangerous, home birth is a safe option, and that women should be given support when they choose home birth. The report asserted that there must be a new professional role for midwives, together with midwifery-managed maternity units. 'We should move as rapidly as possible towards a situation in which midwives ... take full responsibility for the women who are under their care'.

While all this was greeted with enthusiasm by many midwives who found the hierarchical and bureaucratic hospital system frustrating, for some the wind of change blowing through the maternity services was frightening. It threatened security. It wiped out known and trusted parameters of action. It obliterated fine status markers and a tight, tidy structure in which everyone knew their place. Some midwives had a vested interest in retaining the old system of power relations intact, and keeping patients firmly under control. It remains like this today. It would be a disservice to the rebirth of midwifery throughout the world for any advocate of midwife care to fail to acknowledge this with honesty.

As I talked with midwives who reacted like this, I was at first surprised. I have come to realise, however, that there are many who, under the present fragmented system – task-focused rather than woman-focused – in which they serve as agents of crowd control in antenatal clinics, and scuttle around after obstetricians, carrying out their orders and clearing up after them, are tired and overworked, and their job satisfaction has been drained away. Together with childbearing women, they feel caught up in an administrative machine that they cannot influence. They started midwifery with a glow. Now they simply feel exhausted, and any change implies too great a burden of responsibility, too much work, and implies a flexibility that makes them feel insecure.

There were others who were frankly terrified that they would not make the grade. They were probably good 'hands-on' midwives. They knew what to do within the context of the system as it was, but they were frightened that new responsibility would reveal an inadequacy of professional skills, lack of academic learning, and ignorance of the language about midwifery, psychology, relationships and management that has come into use. They might be good midwives, but they, too, saw change as disempowering.

The future for the childbirth services depends on midwives having the courage to create change, to be confident in their skills, to question established systems and methods, and to initiate and undertake their own research. Official committee reports are often a way of shelving issues: 'We set up a committee, deliberated, and produced this report – so that's all that needs to be done'. Yet the Winterton Report was not shelved in this way, if only because of the publicity that it received. Unlike most government reports, it sold like hot cakes.

Midwives actively debated and analysed it, too. A midwifery think-tank was set up at the Nuffield Institute at the University of Leeds, and meetings were held in different parts of the country to explore the issues raised by the report and to design what amounted to new standards of practice and new professional responsibility for midwives. In the Nuffield Institute's publication *Who's Left Holding the Baby? An Organisational Framework for Making the Most of Midwifery Services*,[2] it was proposed that midwives should be 'primary care providers to the 60–70% of women who have normal pregnancies and labour', giving care in the woman's home, in clinics, and in hospitals, and taking responsibility for all the hospital-based care for normal women. The authors of this blueprint for action pointed out that 'although 70% of all babies born in the

United Kingdom are delivered by midwives, the current organisation of maternity care does not allow midwives to function as effectively as they are able'. They recommended a more flexible way of working to avoid 'duplication of effort ... between midwife, general practitioners and hospital doctors (including junior medical staff with little experience) as well as obstetric registrars and consultants'. They proposed that when a woman thought she was pregnant, her first contact should be with a midwife, as is usually the case in The Netherlands, and that no more than six midwives should form a partnership, group practice or team, providing a 24-hour service and taking joint responsibility for 200 cases per annum. They recommended that other hospital-based midwives should provide specialist skills, teach midwifery and medical students, and help the coordination of care between different professional groups.

Some obstetricians reacted with alarm to the Winterton Report, and letters appeared in the *British Medical Journal*; for example, warning that they were the only professionals competent to manage childbirth, since any birth is safe only in retrospect. Shroud-waving of this kind and anecdotes of postpartum haemorrhages following home births attended 30 or 40 years before were to be expected, because the changes in the maternity services that were proposed would limit obstetrician involvement to those pregnancies and births that were abnormal. Normal childbirth was to be conducted by midwives and by the minority of general practitioners (GPs) who chose to give intrapartum care.

Some health administrators welcomed the proposal. One wrote to the *British Medical Journal*, saying: 'It would be surprising if the medical profession did not oppose recommendations to "demedicalise" a service that doctors have tried to monopolise for generations'.[3]

Encouraged by the Winterton Report, the International Home Birth Movement organised a meeting in October 1992 for a small group of people concerned that women should have access to home birth. But as news about it got out, it snowballed into a much larger meeting involving midwives, GPs and others. It was billed as 'Home Birth – A Call for Action' and was attended by over 2000 people.

In 1993, *Changing Childbirth*[4] was published and adopted as government policy. The report of the Expert Maternity Group headed by the parliamentary Under Secretary of State of Health, Baroness Cumberlege, recommended a switch from hospital-oriented services. It stressed that the first principle of the maternity services should be: 'The woman must be the focus of maternity care ... in control of what is happening to her and able to make decisions based on her needs'. Home birth should be a 'real option'. Women should be able to choose where their babies were to be born, and their right to make this choice should be respected. Summarising the recommendations about midwifery, Professor Lesley Page, who was a member of the Expert Group, wrote:[5]

- Every woman should know one midwife who ensures continuity of her midwifery care; the named midwife.
- At least 30% of women should have the midwife as the lead professional.

- Every woman should know the lead professional who has a key role in the planning and provision of her care.
- At least 75% of women should know the person who cares for them during their delivery.
- Midwives should have direct access to some beds in all maternity units.
- At least 30% of women delivered in a maternity unit should be admitted under the management of the midwife.

Changing Childbirth heralded the dawn of mutual understanding, creating a common language, moving toward consensus. Women who give birth, midwives and obstetricians started to talk together and work together in a new way.

Not everyone, of course. The old guard still held its fort with outrage and ferocity, like the witty, urbane senior obstetrician at a conference who referred scathingly to the 'gimmicky demands of a tiny minority' and, referring to water birth, warned the audience against being 'mesmerised by the eccentricities of aquatic fanatics'. Some midwives were still happy to allow women choice in birth only if they stuck to a menu which *they* dictated. Some GPs still struck women off their list for being 'difficult patients' and insisting on home birth. Yet they no longer spoke for the profession and became increasingly isolated. The professional organisations had moved on.

With this, home birth became once again a live issue in Britain. After the powers-that-be ditched home birth in 1970,[6] it was reincorporated into new health service policy, which aimed to give woman-centred care. It was not represented as an 'alternative' option, but as a clear choice for those women who wish it. The media discovered it as a topic, women were discussing it as one of their options with their GPs and midwives, and the rate of home birth, which had sunk to 1%, started to go up again.

At a meeting of the Royal College of Obstetricians and Gynaecologists (RCOG) to discuss *Changing Childbirth*, a senior obstetrician declared that if they resisted the recommendations of this document they would be digging themselves into a corner and 'making total idiots of ourselves'. Another said that obstetricians were damaging the health of low-risk women by insisting on hospital birth for all.

After this meeting *The Times*[7] came out with the headline 'Home birth campaign divides consultants' and *The Independent*[8] with 'Consultant care is no better than midwifery' and 'Opposition to home birth unsuitable for the nineties, obstetrician says', reporting Malcolm Pearce, Consultant Obstetrician and Gynaecologist at St. George's Hospital, who claimed that too many doctors were reluctant to give up their power base in maternity units. His efforts to set up a maternity unit run entirely by midwives was blocked by senior colleagues: 'It is all to do with loss of power; being a consultant is about the numbers of beds and numbers of patients. There is no evidence that consultant care is better than midwifery care, and it is a damn sight more expensive'.

In the same report in *The Independent*, Donald Gibb, Director of Women's Services at King's College Hospital, London, said: 'Women who want home births are treated as selfish – caring only about themselves, not about their babies – and are seen as mad, bad and marginal ... They are not, They are intelligent and sensitive, and want to be involved in a choice about this most important event in their lives'.

The RCOG issued its official response to *Changing Childbirth*, however. It was predictably authoritarian. *Changing Childbirth* spoke of values, philosophy and ethics and at the same time was practical and down-to-earth. The RCOG objected strongly to this and dismissed it as 'rhetoric'.[9] The obstetricians also objected to the term 'lead professional'. It was all right for a midwife to be a 'link', but she must not lead. Ignoring the evidence that already existed from research,[10–17] which suggested that for low-risk women a planned home birth with a midwife made birth as safe as it could be, the RCOG opposed an increase in home births until research had been done into safety, maintaining that delivery is safest in surroundings where expert help was immediately available.[9]

Yet the real problem turned out to be not so much resistance from obstetricians, as resistance from midwives who had received all their training in hospitals, and had no confidence in or understanding of home births. In a commentary on *Changing Childbirth*, Mary Anderson, Consultant at Lewisham Hospital, and member of the Expert Group, remarked that 'Total care by the midwife means that she takes total responsibility, including legal responsibility'.[18] As Wendy Savage, Consultant at the Royal London Hospital, who ran courses for GPs and midwives entitled 'Home Birth for the Hesitant', wrote in a letter to the RCOG, 'What I think is a great challenge is how we are going to encourage midwives to become autonomous after many of them have shown no real interest in practising in an autonomous way, and many of those who wanted to practice in this way have left the profession'.

A new and powerful alliance between organisations of mothers and midwives, striving towards common goals, started to develop. There are only about 850 obstetricians. There are 23,000 midwives, and 700,000 women give birth each year. Women's voices began to be heard – and many were speaking out loud and clear.

But for most women birth remains a medical event. It takes place in hospital, and is thought about almost exclusively in terms of risk. They often do not realise that home birth is possible. Any woman who decides to give birth outside a hospital, at home or in a birth centre, may have to overcome a host of obstacles put in place by the medical system. She is unlikely to get support from family members and friends, either. They say: 'You're very brave!', 'Aren't you worried that something will go wrong?', 'You're being selfish' or 'You're not thinking about the baby'. An extreme example is the Russian grandmother, who was a doctor, who warned that an elective caesarean would be the sensible choice to avoid 'a nasty, fluffy, torn cunt, and be incontinent when you can have a nice little scar, dear'. When her granddaughter in England stuck with her decision to plan a home birth, her grandmother resorted to the final argument of 'wishing both me and the baby to die so that I learned a lesson the hard way'.

Why not a hospital birth room?

'Home from home' and 'birthing' rooms are popping up in hospitals all over the place, in a drive to attract women away from home birth and free-standing birth centres. Hospitals want to budget efficiently, and managers often believe that this can be done only by concentrating resources in one institution, whether or not this is what women want, and although it medicalises all birth, and interventions of every kind, including caesareans, add to the cost. Since most doctors also believe that hospital is the only safe place to have a baby, they tell women, 'You could have everything you want in hospital – music, soft lights, TV, a doula with you, an epidural – and safety, too'. But a woman who wants midwife care and a drug-free birth with no interventions is likely to be transferred to specialised obstetric management as soon as there are any signs that her labour does not conform to the norm imposed by hospital protocol. She is simply wheeled across the corridor, often just because her membranes ruptured early or dilatation is slow. Women who are admitted to hospital in early rather than advanced labour are at greater risk of ending up with a caesarean section. One reason for this is that the clock that monitors active management is set ticking from the moment the woman is admitted. Another reason is that, once in hospital, interventions such as artificial rupture of the membranes and confinement to bed are much more likely than when a woman is labouring at home.[19]

Care in birth centres is much more like that at home. Free-standing, midwife-run birth centres are to be welcomed as an alternative to hospitals and offer women flexibility and freedom. But, once they are established, some midwives want to coax women who ask for home birth into the birth centre, perhaps because professionals feel in control there and work is more convenient on their own base. This has happened in the London area. A birth centre can be superb. But it is not the same as home. Home is where a woman has made her own nest, where she feels most relaxed and can act spontaneously, responding to the hormones rushing through her bloodstream and the power of the contracting uterus, without trying to be on her best behaviour or struggling to put on a good performance. Home is the place where she can be *herself*.

Obstetric interventions, each of which often leads to another, put up the cost of birth. Yet, faced with financial problems, home birth services, although highly valued by mothers, are the first to be cut.[20] Both the North Middlesex Hospitals Home Birth Team, the National Health Service's (NHS's) only specialised service, and small midwife teams, such as the Blue Team in Peterborough, were closed down in spite of calls from the House of Commons Maternity Services Select Committee and the Royal College of Midwives to strengthen home birth services.

In hospital, a normal, healthy woman tends to be treated with all the interventions that are characteristic of high-risk labours. She is seen as a 'not yet ill patient'.[21] And because the birth is managed as if it is high-risk, it often *becomes* high-risk. This is the main reason why caesarean rates are rocketing. In the UK now, approximately one in every four women is delivered by surgery.

In the work I do, everything I have learned from women in countries around the world has convinced me that our medicalised way of birth is not the best way for most women. Yes, there are births where we should be grateful for the support of obstetric skills and high-tech intervention. But for most of us these complicate and impede the normal physiological process and make birth traumatic.

In 1963, when home birth was a normal element in British birth culture, a sociological study of 709 births in the City of Nottingham was conducted by the Newsons.[22] The culture of birth was still social, rather than medical, at that time. But there were ominous indications of change. While 43% of the women in this study who had home births had a woman friend or family member with them in the room at the moment of birth. None of the women who gave birth in hospital had anyone they knew with them.[22]

Subsequently, Margery Tew, a statistician, examined and compared statistics for home and hospital births. Initially, she did this as part of a course teaching statistics to medical students. She thought it would be useful to show how hospital made birth safer. But when she examined the statistics she was astonished to find out that it did not.[23–27]

Julia Allison, a midwife, studied the work of district midwives in 62,444 births in Nottingham during the 24 years between 1948 and 1972. At that time 90% of births at home were attended by the district midwife or her pupil, with no doctor present.[28] She makes the point that 52% of these women did not fulfil the criteria for home birth and would nowadays be considered high risk. The perinatal death rate in the home-booked group was 3 per 1000 births. The perinatal death rate for the hospital-booked group was 75 per 1000 births.

'It has long been assumed that hospital provides a safer environment for women at low risk as well as the high risk mothers. This assumption, however, is not evidence-based'. This statement by two obstetricians, one working in general practice and the other a Professor of Obstetrics, appeared in a 1999 paper in the *British Medical Journal*.[29] Disagreeing, Professor James Drife wrote in to say that women must be warned that home birth is three to four times more dangerous than hospital birth for the baby. He came to this conclusion by comparing home birth outcomes in the USA and Australia with hospital birth outcomes in the UK.[30–33] He also called for research, ignoring the audit of home births in northern England,[34] Olsen's meta-analysis[35] and the *British Medical Journal's* supplement on home birth research in 1996.[36]

Selecting statistics from different countries, as GP obstetrician Gavin Young and paediatrician Edmund Hey quickly pointed out, is a failure to compare like with like: 'It is about as helpful as saying that a man and a dog have an average of three legs'.[37]

In any country the marginalisation of home births makes it dangerous for some women. Punitive attitudes in western Australia have resulted in women who are at known risk having home births because they want to avoid drugs, routine obstetric interventions and unnecessary surgery, and know that they are unlikely to escape these in hospital. When their babies die it is an indictment of the hospital system, rather than of the women who are abused by it.

Birth statistics can only be discussed with validity in a socio-cultural context. Leaping to conclusions about the risk of home birth from figures compiled in Pakistan or Turkey and comparing them with hospital births in the UK, for example, would obviously be ridiculous. Home and hospital births have to be evaluated within a specific healthcare system.

Alison Macfarlane, Rona Campbell and Rona McCandlish, health statisticians, commenting on the studies to which Drife referred, said that there was inconsistency in the definitions of death and the overall groups of birth with which the deaths were compared.[38] Alison Macfarlane and Miranda Mugford's report, *Birth Counts*,[39] confirmed the results of their previous research: that for women who are at low risk, planned home birth is as safe as hospital birth.

The Confidential Enquiry of 1994[40] had already produced some telling statistics, and in meticulous detail: 3896 women had planned home births, 3319 planned hospital births, and 769 women planned a home birth but were transferred to hospital. Those giving birth at home had far fewer interventions:

- 0.2% of those planning home birth had labour induced, compared with 19% of the planned hospital-delivery group
- 7% of home-birth mothers had their membranes artificially ruptured at 4 cm dilatation or less, compared with 25% of those giving birth in hospitals
- 8% of women at home used pethidine compared with 30% of women in hospital
- 24% of those at home used a bath or pool in labour, compared with 8% in hospitals
- women at home usually avoided pain-relieving drugs – less than 10% took any analgesia.

The labours were very different, too. Prolonged labour was reported four times more often and fetal distress three times more often in the hospital births. A woman who planned a hospital delivery was twice as likely to have an operative vaginal delivery or a caesarean section. Women at home were more likely to have an intact perineum, or if they had a tear, had only a first degree laceration. Really severe tears occurred only in hospitals: 48% of women who gave birth at home had an intact perineum, compared with 39% in hospital. Only 4% of women at home received episiotomies, compared with 21% of those in hospital. Women lost less blood when they gave birth at home, although few women in either group actually haemorrhaged. Twice as many in hospital had heavy blood loss and 75% in the home-birth group lost less than 200 ml compared with 65% of hospital-booked women.

Very few babies died in either group, so the numbers of deaths cannot be compared, but the home birth babies were in better condition. Three times as many babies in the planned hospital group suffered fetal distress. Only 4% of babies with home-booked births had Apgar scores below 7 at 1 minute, and only 0.6% at 5 minutes, compared with 9% and 1%, respectively, of those booked for hospital deliveries. In the home group, 13% of babies were resuscitated, usually simply being given a whiff of oxygen, compared with 28% of the hospital group.

Olsen's meta-analysis, based on research studies into planned home births in industrialised countries where there is a modern healthcare system, examined 24,092 home births, and matched them with births to other low-risk pregnant women planning birth in hospitals.[35] Significantly fewer women who planned a home birth were induced, had an episiotomy, or ended up with an operative vaginal delivery or a caesarean section. They were less likely to have a bad perineal tear and their babies were in better condition at birth. The conclusion is: 'Home birth is an acceptable alternative to hospital confinement for selected pregnant women, and leads to reduced medical interventions'. Although the authors stated that 'There is no evidence to support the claim that the safest policy is for all women to give birth in hospital', as Chamberlain pointed out in the 1994 Confidential Enquiry: 'It seems clear that whatever the evidence many leading obstetricians are unlikely to move away from their position of advocating hospital delivery for all women'.[40]

Women in hospital said that the most important thing for them about being in hospital was that it made them feel safe. Yet safety is not the only issue. Birth is a major life event and it is much easier to start out on mothering when the experience brings fulfilment and triumph. An unhappy woman may find it difficult to enjoy building a relationship with her new baby, and face problems in breastfeeding. In the study,[40] 80% of the home birth mothers breastfed within the first 48 hours, compared with 58% of the hospital mothers. Home birth mothers were less likely to have backache, headache, perineal pain or tiredness. Many women said they had dreadful postnatal care in hospital, so they were glad to get home. An important element in women's experiences of home birth was that they were free of stress and in control of their own territory. No woman who gave birth at home said that she felt she was not in control.

The National Childbirth Trust published a report based on evidence from Maternity Service Liaison Committees all over the country, which showed that more than 50% of doctors opposed home births and over 50% of women were cared for by several midwives they had never met before.[41] There are indications that some women may have no option if they want a home birth but to 'go it alone' with a neighbour or family member to help.

GPs are the gate-keepers to the place of birth. Some warn women that they may haemorrhage to death, or their babies may die or be brain damaged, if they insist on home birth. I hear every week from women who are asked 'Do you want to have a dead baby? How could you ever forgive yourself?' They are told, 'It's not safe to have a first baby at home' or 'You might bleed to death'. GPs can strike a recalcitrant patient off their register without any further explanation.

Alternatively, they can play along with her until at the end of pregnancy they announce that her blood pressure is up or the baby is too large, or too small, or in a difficult position, without producing evidence for this.

Lorna Davies, a midwife in Essex, asked members of the UK Midwifery List, set up by the Association of Radical Midwives in 1999, for information about why home births were not allowed. Responses came from midwives, students and mothers. The list of reasons given is shown in Table 12.1.[42] She says that some of these reasons were recurrent, but she chose to include them once only.

Table 12.1 Why home births are not allowed

Current pregnancy
- Baby is too small
- Baby is too big
- Woman is too old (age 37)
- Woman is too young (age 16)
- Too little amniotic fluid
- Too much amniotic fluid
- Baby is too early (36 weeks + 6 days)
- Baby is too late (1 week overdue)
- Untried pelvis – may be allowed next time
- Untested pelvis
- Fourth pregnancy
- You've more than three children already, so might haemorrhage
- I don't match the 'criteria' for being 'permitted' a home birth as I am having my fifth baby
- You've had two babies already and your uterus is knackered
- Gestational diabetes
- Breech baby
- Blood pressure too high (on one occasion after I had rushed from work to attend an antenatal appointment)
- You have had high blood pressure, if you want to put your baby at risk go ahead!

Obstetric history
- Previous placental abruption (for a woman who hadn't had one!)
- Previous section
- You had a borderline test for gestational diabetes in your last pregnancy, so although there's no evidence of GD this time, you can't have a home birth
- How about 'not with your history' when pregnant with baby number 4 following one vaginal breech, one SVD and one ventouse
- They had had a 28 weeker previously
- Previous ectopic pregnancy
- First baby died 29 days post-birth due to large tumour. Second baby born fine after normal pregnancy and birth. Now pregnant again, and midwife phoned re. booking. Woman explains about first baby, and is wanting home birth. Midwife response is 'one dead baby means no home birth'

Medical history
- History of depression
- You are diabetic, if you want to kill your baby go ahead!
- Heart murmur
- Partially sighted
- Family history
- My mother has type II diabetes

Social factors
- Accommodation not spacious enough

Table 12.1 continued

- Terraced house (neighbours might hear)
- Live in a council flat
- Husband with a history of depression
- Woman who wanted to give birth on a houseboat was told that it was not possible because the mid-wife might fall off the towpath into the canal
- Body mass index (BMI) too great
- Husband too big

Staffing issues
- We don't have enough staff to cover a home birth
- There are three other women due at the same time so you might have to come in (apparently in this particular area there are always '3' other home births booked)
- If we don't have enough midwives on, you'll have to come in on the night
- Had turned down any scans, so midwives would not feel happy being at the delivery as 'they wouldn't know what they were dealing with'
- You can't have a home birth because we haven't delivered your home birth pack yet

- You'd be taking two midwives away from the hospital
- Labouring women in hospital their first priority
- The midwife said she couldn't because it takes 4 weeks to organise a birth pack (gas and air, etc.)
- Multiparous woman was told she would have to come into labour ward when she had SROM as they did not want to wake the community midwife up
- Lots of midwives likely to be off sick with colds around that time (February)

Miscellaneous
- No one trained to do waterbirth
- We don't do waterbirths (they are not natural)
- Have to get an electrician out from hospital to check your wiring
- Worried I might sue if something went wrong at home
- You can't have any pain relief at home
- Baby may be born flat
- GP not delivered a baby in years
- I would have to find a GP who would agree to it

SROM, spontaneous rupture of membranes; SVD, spontanous vaginal delivery

Women are also told that they are being 'selfish' in taking up a midwife's time at home, when she could be overseeing three or four births simultaneously on the labour ward. The midwife shortage is acute. Many midwives leave the profession because of low job satisfaction. Letters are sent out by Health Trusts instructing pregnant women who have already booked for home birth that they may have to come into hospital. In some cases women have been told this as late as 39 weeks' gestation. A woman who has planned a home birth may have even started labour, when a midwife visits and follows instructions from management to 'encourage' her to go into hospital.

Resources are drained out of community care and injected into acute services. The Royal College of Midwives advises Trusts to employ additional bank (reserve) or agency staff on the labour ward, to release midwives to attend home births and to contract home-birth services out to independent midwives.[43] It goes on to say that: 'The RCM accepts that there may be emergency situations where the only way to ensure the safety of all women is to focus resources on a hospital birth service. However, this should be treated as a significant breach of good practice and should be reviewed in order to minimise the chances of it happening again'.

In 2004 a midwife was sacked in Peterborough, where there is a home-birth rate of only 0.5%, for 'gross insubordination' because he attended a woman who was having a planned home birth when the Trust had decided to suspend services. Another woman, who had also arranged a home birth with him, was visited by a supervisor and persuaded to go into hospital.

Paul Beland had been a manager's thorn in the flesh for some time. In 1999 he challenged Peterborough Trust's right to charge for attendance at antenatal classes, and wrote to Alan Milburn, the Secretary for State for Health and the professional journals. This stimulated publicity in the national media. A Department of Health spokesperson reiterated: 'The Secretary of State has made it clear that charges of this kind are not acceptable'.

Mr Milburn called on the Chief Executive of the Trust to explain why they had ever considered such a proposal. Yet other trusts were already charging. Mount Vernon and Watford and St. Albans and Hemel Hempstead had been charging £50 for a course of antenatal classes for many years. They were forced to stop the practice too. Paul Beland wrote in the *British Journal of Midwifery* that, because Peterborough Trust had overspent by more than £1 million, it was at risk of having an outside management team appointed and suggested: 'It may be the threat to senior managerial careers that stimulated the reckless search for cost cutting and fund raising schemes'.[44, 45]

Paul had already written an article in the *British Journal of Midwifery* 3 years before, quoting rule 40(1) of the Midwives Rules and Code of Practice:

> *The midwife should not refuse to continue to provide care for a woman on the basis of where the woman wishes the birth to take place ... If mutually acceptable arrangements cannot be agreed, the midwife should not withdraw care, thereby potentially placing the woman at risk of delivering unattended ... If her [the mother's] decision is to continue with the planned home birth, the midwife should not withdraw care.[46]*

He went on to say:

> *In effect, any attempt by NHS trusts to deny a woman a home birth service has the status of a bluff, depending on intimidated women not calling it.*

On the BBC radio programme *Woman's Hour*, the head of midwifery services at Peterborough claimed that women in the Peterborough area do not want home birth.[47] She implied that services were withdrawn because the demand was low. As Belinda Phipps, Director of the National Childbirth Trust, pointed out in the same programme: 'You wouldn't say that because few people need a blood transfusion you shouldn't have a service'. A spokesperson for the Nursing and Midwifery Council stressed that women have the right to give birth at home and it is a midwife's duty to support them.[48]

Frances Day-Stirk of the Royal College of Midwives says: 'Care should follow the woman'. She believes that when units are short-staffed, heads of midwifery should have the courage to say: '"We won't do an elective caesarean today. There is a woman having a home birth". At present the focus is exclusively on acute care'.

Trusts no longer accept responsibility to provide a community midwifery service. Care is fragmented and women are being directed to hospital whether they like it or not. The Audit Commission's report, published in 1997, concluded that it is a matter of luck, depending on where they live, whether women can get a home birth. There is lip-service to the idea of choice, but it usually does not include home birth.[49]

Trusts have not had a statutory duty to provide a domiciliary birth service since the NHS was reorganised in the 1970s. By an oversight, provision for this was omitted. Yet it is government policy that women have the right to give birth at home and it is the midwife's professional responsibility to attend a woman in labour wherever she is.[39] The only exception to women's legal right to home birth is if they are admitted to hospital under the Mental Health Act. The result is that midwives are confused by contradictory guidance and there is a head-on collision between women seeking home birth and a centralised, rigid, hierarchical and hospital-dominated medical system.

But this is not the whole story. Every NHS Trust is insured against clinical negligence. The insurance company lays down rules. The names of their medical advisors are not open to public scrutiny. Nor do we know on what research evidence, if any, they base their regulations. So, ultimately, the protocols are dictated by faceless individuals who are invisible and unaccountable to the users of the NHS.

Even when a woman is booked for a home birth, she may not know who in a team of anything up to 11 midwives will attend her in labour. It is often someone whom she has never met before. Midwives do not, as a rule, get any training in home birth. A midwife who lacks confidence communicates her anxiety to the mother, and may put her under pressure to accept transfer to hospital. She insists on this because the membranes have ruptured early, or dilatation is not fast enough, and may persuade her that the baby is 'in distress', without any evidence of it on the labour chart.

This is occurring in spite of a strong statement by the Royal College of Midwives that: 'Home birth can no longer be regarded as a special privilege for a fringe minority – it should be understood as integral and mainstream to any modern maternity service'.[43]

Midwives are cogs in a medical system that is based on hospitals and permeated by a philosophy of care that is focused on pathology. Yet some areas of the country have got it right and enable women to have home birth. Midwifery organisation is superb in the Torquay area of Devon, and around Bath, Scunthorpe, Blackburn and Shrewsbury. The Albany Group Practice in London has a home birth rate of 43%.[50] In Torbay, a community midwife attends a woman in labour at home, if she plans to have a home birth, and the mother can decide whether or not she wants to go into hospital as labour progresses. Midwives have direct phone access to consultant obstetricians. The result is that the home birth rate in this part of the south-west is 11–12%, five times higher than the national average. This system reduces the number of women entering hospital in early labour who go on to have multiple interventions and often end up with a caesarean section. Far from being short of midwives, Torbay has a waiting list of midwives who are eager to work there. Other hospitals that willingly provide a home-birth service find no difficulty in attracting midwives, too. These are the places where midwives want to work. A report from the Royal College of Midwives makes it clear that midwives prefer hospitals that do not have a conveyor belt system.[51]

The creation of the NHS was a brave and splendid revolution. As a child, I remember my mother's excitement. She had been a midwife and had also worked in one of England's first family planning clinics. She used to talk about the distress surrounding pregnancy and birth for many impoverished women who were unable to have any control over their reproductive lives. They saved money in a tin on the kitchen shelf so that their children could get medical care, but could not afford it themselves. Together with the improved nutrition that came about as the result of food rationing during and after the Second World War, the NHS changed the health of a nation.

Government policy on birth initiated in 1998[52] seemed to herald another revolution, and for the first time promised woman-centred care. But the changes made have not matched the fine talk. The system is fettered by fortress-like management structures and insensitive, defensive attitudes. We may have reached the stage where legal action is necessary. Barbara Hewson, the barrister who appealed against court-enforced caesarean sections, and won a landmark case, considers that home birth is a question of human rights.

Kafka said: 'Every revolution evaporates and leaves behind it only the slime of a new bureaucracy'. I believe that the birth revolution has to be continually recreated if we are to improve the quality of childbirth for women and their babies everywhere.

Why do some women want home birth?

Women rarely feel they need to justify the choice of a hospital birth. Those who opt for hospital tend to think of it as the normal way to have a baby. If asked why they are going into hospital they may say that it is safer for the baby and themselves, they can get an epidural there, and that since expertise and equipment is based at the hospital, they will have speedy access to skills and technology. Some say that birth is messy and this is why they prefer it to take place in hospital. Some say that their male partners insist that hospital is best, and that the men could not cope with home birth.

A large proportion of women who have given birth previously in hospital seek a home birth because the hospital birth was distressing. They hope that it will avoid a style of birth in which they are confronted by strangers, denied information and choice, treated like a 'lump of meat', and feel completely out of control. One woman, who questioned the need for induction of labour, described how the obstetric registrar told her: 'When I go to the garage, I do not tell the mechanic how to fix my car'.

A study reveals that women in Sweden who choose to give birth at home or a birth centre want to feel in control and think that this is much more likely at home or in a midwife-run birth centre. They want to make their own decisions, manage without pharmacological pain relief, have a known midwife, and give birth naturally. They see birth as a social, rather than a medical, event. The authors of this study conclude that: 'If women had free choice of place of birth the home birth rate in Sweden would be 10 times higher and the 20 largest hospitals would need to have birth centers'.[53]

Women who call me often talk about why they seek a home birth. Their main concerns are described below.

To handle birth without drugs

One reason is that the women do not want to be dosed to the eyeballs with drugs. All anaesthetic and analgesic drugs cross the placenta to the fetus. I have heard an obstetric anaesthetist describe the placenta as 'a sump for drugs'. Drug transfer is flow-dependent. Fetal plasma has a lower pH than maternal plasma, so the drug *concentrates* in the fetus.

Pethidine is a weak analgesic but a strong respiratory depressant. After a single dose there is a higher concentration in the fetus than in the mother, and it can be detected in the newborn baby for 62 hours.

An epidural can bring blessed relief from pain and does not produce respiratory depression. When given by an experienced anaesthetist it is usually safe. But epidurals often have side-effects for the mother and the baby: 15% of mothers and babies develop fever during labour. The baby may be taken to the special-care nursery for investigation and tests to discover if it has septicaemia. The mother's blood pressure may drop suddenly when the epidural is given, and this reduces the amount of oxygen passing through the placenta to the baby. So other drugs have to be available to raise the mother's blood pressure again. Delivery may be by forceps or ventouse because the tone of the pelvic floor muscles is lost, the head gets stuck in the wrong position, and the mother cannot push the baby out.

The vaginal operative delivery rate is four times higher in women who have epidurals than in those who do not, and the caesarean rate is twice as high.[54–57]

To give birth without intervention

Each intervention in childbirth has a knock-on effect that can be positive or negative. It may help to support the physiology of normal labour, or disrupt it so that there is a cascade of further interventions. There is evidence that induction of labour leads to other interventions, including greater need for pain-killing drugs. One study showed that induction more than doubles the likelihood that delivery will be by caesarean section.[58]

Continuous fetal monitoring is also associated with other interventions, including instrumental delivery and caesarean section.[59–62] The problem is that fetal distress is often diagnosed when it is not present.[63] In UK hospitals the trend is towards routine admission cardiotocography (CTG) for 20 minutes. This has the effect of classifying a large group of women as having abnormalities when, in fact, labour is normal and the baby is fine. In one study, 32% of print-outs were defined as unsatisfactory, and the women went on to have continuous CTG.[64]

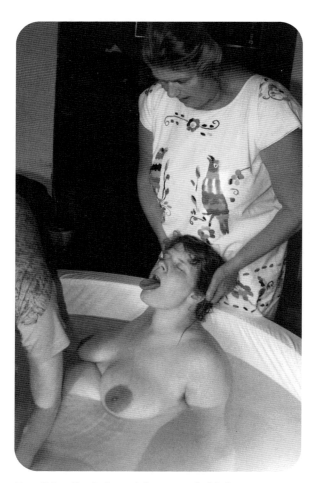

Breathing the baby out for a gentle birth

Labour can be disturbed by midwifery interventions, too, some of which have been made for many years without any analysis of their effect. As one midwife teacher expresses it: 'Decades of repetitive performance of asking a woman to get on a bed, or asking her to push, have had the effect of making such interventions invisible'.[65] Amniotomy, for example, is often used routinely, and injections of pethidine are part of normal midwifery practice.

In the USA multiple interventions are the norm. The First National Survey of Women's Child-bearing Experiences reveals that 93% of women had continuous electronic fetal monitoring, 86% an intravenous drip, 74% of those who gave birth vaginally were expected to lie on their backs while pushing the baby out, 67% had artificial oxytocin to start or to stimulate uterine contractions, 63% had epidurals, 58% had a hand inserted into the uterus after birth, 55% had their membranes artificially ruptured, 52% had a catheter in the bladder, and 52% had suturing to repair an episiotomy or tear. Less than 1% of women gave birth without such interventions, and nearly all these came from the less than 1% home births in the sample.[66]

To enable the baby to have a smooth and gentle introduction to the world

Newborn babies can see and hear. They look around and fix their eyes on the nearest interesting face. They startle if they hear loud noises, and turn towards the sound of the mother's voice, because they heard it when inside her body.

All this is delayed if the baby is crying so much that other stimuli are shut out, or is so drugged that he or she cannot respond to anything. At birth, babies often cry for about 5 minutes. A very heavily drugged baby feels floppy and may only whimper, or may not cry at all. A distressed baby may cry until it is exhausted. In general, babies who have received analgesic drugs from their mothers cry longer than babies of mothers who have received no drugs.[67–69]

A newborn baby who has not been dosed with medication in the maternal bloodstream is in an ideal neurophysiological state to start out on the exciting task of getting to know its mother and to breastfeed.[67]

Given time, and in a relaxed environment, a baby will spontaneously creep up towards the breast,[69] and then starts to root, turning its head from side to side, mouth open and searching for the nipple. It uses its hands as well as its mouth. Immediately after birth the hands are relaxed, but after a few minutes they start to explore. The baby sucks its fingers and strokes and massages the breast, licks it, and, in its own time, latches on and sucks.[70] This process usually takes about an hour, during which time the baby should not be disturbed or taken away. There is no hurry to weigh, bath or dress a newborn. It is much easier to create a birth setting in which babies can behave spontaneously, and mothers can behave more spontaneously, too, at home than in hospital.

The mother responds to the baby's stimulation with a rush of oxytocin, which causes the uterus to contract and expel the placenta and makes her nipples erect, ready for feeding. She is excited, and touches the baby, first with her finger tips, then with the whole palm, and enfolds the baby in the crook of her arm. She cannot take her eyes off her baby, who stares and searches her face, fascinated by her eyes and mouth, and the movements as she smiles and speaks. A new relationship is unfolding. Two people are getting to know each other.

To have a midwife they know

Women seeking a home birth do not just want a 'named midwife' or 'continuity of care' offered by a team of midwives whose faces and names they struggle to recognise. They want a midwife whom they come to know during pregnancy, and who by the time the baby is due has become a close friend.

There is a world of difference between knowing your midwife's name and phone number or meeting a large group of midwives any two of whom might attend you in labour, and having a special relationship with someone you like and trust, and who really knows you. It is reasonable to be cared for by two to four midwives working together, but not to have to confront a group the size of a football team.

Unfortunately, when women are booked for a home birth they are often told that they will be cared for by a team of midwives, or that someone might come out from hospital when labour starts whom they have never before met, and that even this cannot be guaranteed: if the labour ward is short staffed, home birth is impossible and they must come in.

This leaves many pregnant women feeling very unsure of what is going to happen. They are up against an administrative structure that is rigid and implacable. However reassuring the individuals they meet, they cannot fight the system.

So what may have been the priority reason that leads a woman to choose home birth – personal, sensitive, and usually woman-to-woman care (for a small percentage ofmidwives are men) – her choice is denied her.

If she is seeking a personal relationship with the midwife, it is sensible to try to find a midwife who has responsibility for her own case load. This system operates in only a few areas within the NHS. It is what independent midwives offer. But, because these work outside the NHS, they have to be paid for.

To be free to move around

The medical management of childbirth that was introduced in the 20th century confined women to bed, because this was the easiest place for a doctor to keep an eye on them, and they could maintain their modesty by being covered in bedding. Whereas prior to this time it was taken for granted that women in labour were upright, moved around, and used a rope from the rafters, window ledges and a table or chair to get into comfortable positions, once a doctor was in charge, even in home births, the requirements of medical supervision, together with modesty, dictated that a woman should be in bed and under the covers. In her own home a woman can move freely, supporting herself in any position she chooses, using furniture with which she is familiar. She does not need special equipment to stand, squat or kneel.

Movement is almost invariably restricted in hospital, since the mother is harpooned to electronic equipment, and perhaps an intravenous drip. There is no question of this happening in the environment of home. She can squat in front of a chair, the children's toy box, be on all fours on the floor, or in the bath or on the bed, lean against the kitchen units or a window ledge, rock her pelvis, knees spread, against the dining room table or a desk, or over a hammock and do a gentle belly dance with strong, flexible support – any of these, and more.

In hospital, birth tends to be much more static, especially once the second stage is reached. The main participants are positioned as if in a tableau and according to their status in the hierarchy. The senior obstetrician or midwife in charge stands at the end of the delivery table or bed between the woman's legs. Others are grouped around, with her partner up at her head. She may look down and see a man's face between her legs. He may be a total stranger.

To avoid hospital cross-infection

Streptococcus B is the main cause of neonatal sepsis. Mothers and babies are especially at risk when interventions take place that entail early artificial rupture of the membranes, frequent pelvic examinations, insertion of foreign bodies, such as catheters and other instruments, into the vagina, and the crowding of women together under insanitary conditions, with midwives caring for several women simultaneously.

Home birth is a social, rather than a medical, model of birth

Other reasons for choosing home birth are to do with human values. Birth and the events surrounding it have traditionally been a domestic ritual and female celebration. In the Christian calendar women organise making pancakes on Shrove Tuesday, hot cross buns at Easter, and family get togethers at Christmas, so in the past women planned and choreographed what was to happen during birth and the lying-in, and cooked special dishes to keep up the labouring woman's strength, and to celebrate after the birth. Childbirth took place in women's space, not a male-dominated institution. At all levels of society women gathered, bringing their charms, herbs and 'simples' to support the mother.

Even when a doctor attended, but birth still took place at home, it was expected that other women would be present to help. Doctors complained that they could do nothing without the women's agreement. It was the move from home to hospital that finally got rid of the group of women companions.

At home birth is a social process, rather than a medical crisis. It is an intimate and domestic event, and the parameters of time are quite different from those of hospital births. The medical model defines childbirth in terms of three stages: the first stage in which the cervix dilates to 10 cm, the second stage in which the baby is expelled, and the third stage in which the other products of conception

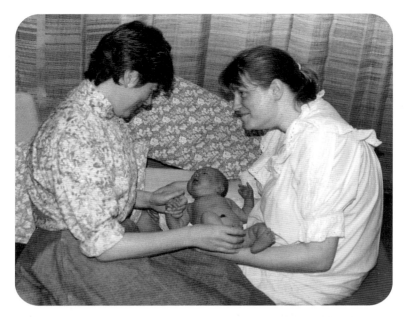

At home postnatal care is part of a continuous relationship with the midwife

(placenta and membranes) are expelled. Birth is segmented into specific periods of time, and the time taken for each phase is noted on a record sheet.

A holistic view of birth time does not mean that the midwife is neglectful of or casual about the passage of time or the efficiency of uterine function, but that she assesses it in terms of the woman's personality, her behaviour, and relationships and the setting in which the birth is taking place.

With the switch to hospital, birth became a medical drama, unfolding as if on a stage or at an altar. The lighting is often harsh and inflexible, and the mother may be under the full glare of fluorescent lights, more suited to a fast-food joint or fish and chip shop.

Imagine being told to make love in the setting of the hospital delivery room typical of almost anywhere in the world today. There is a hard, narrow bed in the centre of the room, a trolley with metal instruments, and a pervasive odour of antiseptics. A clock is on the wall opposite the delivery table and there is a spy-hole window in the door, which opens and closes as complete strangers pop in and out to have a look or to relay a piece of information about what is happening in another room down the corridor.

Or try enjoying a meal in a laboratory surrounded by steel instruments while harpooned to electronic equipment. Specialists in gastroenterology watch and time you, rate your performance, write up detailed notes, and exhort you to try harder and swallow faster.

Our bodies tend to function more effectively when we are in a familiar environment that we ourselves can control, and in which we can relax and behave spontaneously. The challenge to hospitals is to create an environment in which this is possible for *all* women, whether low or high risk.

References

1. Health Committee 1992 Report on the maternity services, vol 1 [Winterton Report]. London: HMSO

2. Ball JA, Flint C, Garvey M, et al 1992 Who's left holding the baby? An organisational framework for making the most of midwifery services. Leeds: Nuffield Institute, University of Leeds

3. Schatzberger P 1992. Maternity services [letter]. BMJ 304(6838):1382–1383

4. Department of Health 1993 Changing childbirth. Part 1: Report of the expert maternity group. London: HMSO

5. Page L. Changing childbirth. MIDIRS Midwifery Digest 1993; 3(4):385–387.

6. Department of Health. Central Health Services Council 1970 Domiciliary midwifery and maternity bed needs. Report of a sub-committee of the Standing Maternity and Midwifery Advisory Committee [Peel Report]. London: HMSO

7. Home birth campaign divides consultants. The Times, 13 October 1993

8. Consultant care is no better than midwifery. The Independent, 13 October 1993. Opposition to home birth unsuitable for the nineties, obstetrician says. The Independent, 13 October 1993

9. Dunlop W 1993 Changing childbirth. Commentary II. British Journal of Obstetrics and Gynaecology 100(12):1072–1074

10. Damstra-Wijmenga SMI 1984 Home confinement: the positive results in Holland. Journal of the Royal College of General Practitioners 34(265):425–430

11. Tew M, Damstra-Wijmenga SM 1991 Safest birth attendants: recent Dutch evidence. Midwifery 7(2):55–63

12. Caplan M, Madeley RJ 1985 Home deliveries in Nottingham 1980–81. Public Health 99(5):307–313

13. Howe KA 1988 Home births in south-west Australia. Medical Journal of Australia 149(6):296–302

14. Tew M 1985 Place of birth and perinatal mortality. Journal of the Royal College of General Practitioners 35(277):390–394

15. Ford C, Iliffe S, Franklin O 1991 Outcome of planned home births in an inner city practice. BMJ 303(6816):1517–1519

16. Campbell R, MacFarlane A, Cavenagh S 1991 Choice and chance in low risk maternity care. BMJ 303(6816):1487–1488

17. Campbell R, MacFarlane A 1987 Where to be born? The debate and the evidence. Oxford: National Perinatal Epidemiology Unit

18. Anderson M 1993 Changing childbirth. Commentary I. British Journal of Obstetrics and Gynaecology 100(12):1071–1072

19. Leyshon L 1999 Integrating caseloads across a whole service: the Torbay model. MIDIRS Midwifery Digest 14(1 Suppl):9–11

20. Newburn M 2003 Reconfiguring maternity services. Views of user representatives. London: National Childbirth Trust

21. Walsh D 2001 Birth as risky behaviour: reflections on risk management. MIDIRS Midwifery Digest 13(4):545–549

22. Newson J, Newson E 1963 Patterns of infant care in an urban community. London: Penguin

23. Tew M 1978 Intended place of delivery and perinatal outcome. BMJ 1(6120): 1139–1140

24. Tew M 1979 The safest place of birth. Lancet i(8131):1388–1390

25. Tew M 1985 Place of birth and perinatal mortality. Journal of the Royal College of General Practitioners 35(277):390–394

26. Tew M 1986 Do obstetric intranatal interventions make birth safer? British Journal of Obstetrics and Gynaecology 93(7):659–674

27. Tew M 1995 Safer childbirth, 2nd edn. London: Chapman & Hall

28. Allison J 1996 Delivered at home. London: Chapman & Hall

29. Zander L, Chamberlain G 1999 ABC of labour care: place of birth. BMJ 318(7185): 721–723

30. Drife JO 1999 Data on babies' safety during hospital births are being ignored [letter]. BMJ 319(7215):1008

31. Anderson RE, Murphy PA 1995 Outcomes of 11,788 planned home births attended by certified nurse-midwives. Journal of Nurse Midwifery 40(6):483–492

32. Murphy PA, Fullerton J 1988 Outcomes of intended home births in nurse-midwifery practice. Obstetrics and Gynecology 92(3):461–470

33. Bastian H, Keirse MJ, Lancaster PA 1998 Perinatal death associated with planned home births in Australia. BMJ 317(7155):384–388

34. Northern Region Perinatal Mortality Survey Coordinating Group 1996 Collaborative survey of perinatal loss in planned and unplanned home births. BMJ 313(7068):1302–1306

35. Olsen O 1997 Meta-analysis of the safety of home birth. Birth 24(1):4–13

36. Davies J, Hey E, Reid W, et al 1996 Prospective regional study of planned home births. BMJ 313(7068):1302–1306

37. Young G, Hey E 2000 Choosing between home and hospital delivery. Home birth in Britain can be safe [letter]. BMJ 319(7215):798

38. Macfarlane A, Campbell R, McCandlish R 1999 Data on babies' home births are being ignored. Response to Drife J. Data on babies' hospital births are being ignored [letter]. BMJ 319(1008)

39. Macfarlane A, Mugford M 2000 Care of mothers and babies. Birth counts: statistics of pregnancy and childbirth, 2nd edn. Oxford: National Perinatal Epidemiology Unit

40. Chamberlain G, Wraight A, Crowley P 1997 Home births: the report of the 1994 confidential enquiry National Birthday Trust Fund. Carnforth: Parthenon

41. Newburn M 2003 Reconfiguring maternity services. Views of user representatives. London: National Childbirth Trust

42. Davies L 2004 'Allowed' shouldn't be allowed! MIDIRS Midwifery Digest 14(2):151–156

43. Royal College of Midwives 2002 Position Paper 25. Home birth. Available at: http://www.rcm.org.uk/data/info_centre/data/position_papers.htm (accessed November 2004)

44. Beland P 2000 Antenatal class charges: are they harebrained proposals? British Journal of Midwifery 8(1)

45. Milburn A 1999 Daily Mail, 26 November 1999

46. Beland P 2001 Individual Trusts are impeding home birth, not the UKCC. British Journal of Midwifery 9(1)

47. Woman's Hour, BBC Radio 4, 27 August 2004

48. Midwife guidelines to be reviewed. Peterborough Evening Telegraph, 26 August 2004. Available at: http://www.peterboroughtoday.co.uk (accessed November 2004)

49. Audit Commission 1997 First class delivery: improving maternity services in England and Wales. Abingdon: Audit Commission Publications

50. Sandall J, Davies J, Warwick C 2001 Evaluation of the Albany Midwifery Practice: final report. Available at: http://www.kcl.ac.uk/nmvc/resrearch/project/mwhrg/albany_final_rpt.pdf

51. Kirkham M 2004 Why do midwives leave? London: RCM Publications. Available at: http://www.rcm-publications.co.uk (accessed November 2004)

52. United Kingdom Central Council 1998 Midwives' rules and code of practice. London: UKCC, pp 27–28

53. Hildingsson I, Waldenstrom U, Radestad I 2003 Swedish women's interest in home birth and in-hospital birth center care. Birth 30(1):11–22

54. Findley I, Chamberlain G 1999 ABC of labour care: relief of pain. BMJ 318(7188):927–930

55. Goer H 1999 The thinking woman's guide to a better birth. New York: Penguin Putman

56. MacArthur C, Weeks S 1995 Epidural anaesthesia and low back pain after delivery: a prospective cohort study. BMJ 311(7016):1336–1339

57. Thorp JA, Hu DA, Albin RM, et al 1993 The effect of intrapartum epidural analgesia on nulliparous labor: a randomized, controlled, prospective trial. American Journal of Obstetrics and Gynecology 169(4):851–858

58. Seyb ST, Berka RJ, Socol ML, et al 1999 Risk of cesarean delivery with elective induction of labor at term in nulliparous women. Obstetrics and Gynaecology 94(4):600–607

59. Haverkamp AD, Thompson HE, McFee JG, et al 1976 The evaluation of continuous fetal heart rate monitoring in high-risk pregnancy. American Journal of Obstetrics and Gynecology 125(3):310–317

60. Renou P, Chang A, Anderson I, et al 1976 Controlled trial of fetal intensive care. American Journal of Obstetrics and Gynecology 126(4):470–476

61. Vintzileos AM, Antsaklis A, Varvarigos I, et al 1993 A randomised trial of intrapartum electronic fetal heart rate monitoring versus intermittent auscultation. American Journal of Obstetrics and Gynecology 81(6):899–907

62. Thacker SB, Stroup DF 2000 Continuous electronic heart rate monitoring for fetal assessment during labor. Cochrane Library, Issue 2. Oxford: Update Software

63. Ecker JL, Chen KT, Cohen AP, et al 2001 Increased risk of cesarean delivery with advancing maternal age: indications and associated factors in nulliparous women. American Journal of Obstetrics and Gynecology 185(4):883–887

64. Impey L, Reynolds M, MacQuillan K, et al 2003 Admission cardiotocography: a randomised controlled trial. Lancet 361(9356):465–470

65. Anderson A 2002 Peeling back the layers: a new look at midwifery interventions. MIDIRS Midwifery Digest 12(2):208

66. Declercq ER, Sakala C, Corry MP, et al 2002 Listening to mothers: report of the first national US survey of women's childbearing experiences. Conducted for the Maternity Center Association by Harris Interactive, Rochester, NY

67. Ransjo-Arvidson AB, Matthiesen AS, Lilja G, et al 2001 Maternal analgesia during labor disturbs newborn behavior: effects on breastfeeding, temperature and crying. Birth 28(1):5–12

68. Sepkoski CM, Lester BM, Ostheimer GW, et al 1992 The effects of maternal epidural anesthesia on neonatal behavior during the first month. Developments in Medicine and Child Neurology 34(12):1072–1080

69. Belsey EM, Rosenblatt DB, Lieberman BA, et al 1981 The influence of maternal analgesia on neonatal behaviour. I. Pethidine. British Journal of Obstetrics and Gynaecology 188:398–406

70. Matthiesen AS, Ransjo-Arvidson AB, Nissen E, et al 2001 Postpartum maternal oxytocin release by newborns: effects of infant hand massage and sucking. Birth 28(1):13–19

13

Waterbirth

How waterbirth started

Although it is sometimes thought that waterbirth has a long history, evidence for it in the past and for birth in water in other cultures is sparse. Mostly women have sought out, or had built for them, a secluded, dark place, a room by the stove in temperate climates, a fern-cushioned space in the bush, a mossy enclosure, or a sand- or fur-carpeted tent.

In New Zealand there is one Maori mountain tribe in which local tradition has it that birth took place in a sacred river, and women in many Pacific island cultures went down to the shore to give birth beside the water or in the shallows, delivered the placenta in the water, and bathed postpartum. But beyond that, accounts are few and far between.[1]

In general, water has been in short supply and too precious to be used in a tub for birth. Like eating the placenta, waterbirth is more likely to be encountered in California, or, for that matter, in Kensington, than in traditional cultures. It is part of a new birth culture that challenges the dominant medical system of birth. It does not need to be validated by tradition.

Certainly, birth in which the woman is *immersed* in water is a recent innovation, and the first records come from Russia, where Igor Charkovsky, originally a boat builder, who was working in the shaman tradition, started a waterbirth movement in the 1970s. Women went to the Black Sea with their families and midwives to give birth in the rocky coves. This was in dramatic contrast to the regimentation, routine enemas and pubic shaves, and the exercise of rigid medical authority, typical of most Russian hospitals.[2]

Water was introduced for the baby, not the mother, by Frederick LeBoyer in France.[3] He had a bath waiting for the baby at birth, whom he cradled in his hands in the water, the head not submerged. He claimed that it was of benefit to the neonate because the transition to an environment in which it had to breathe air became gentler and slower. The focus was on the benefit to the baby.

Subsequently, Dr Michel Odent, a French surgeon who questioned why he was required to perform so many caesarean sections in a small state-run clinic in Pithiviers, introduced pools as a means of facilitating the mother's relaxation and ability to cut out extraneous influences, so that she could trust her instincts and work harmoniously with her body. Beginning with a children's paddling pool, he later had custom-made birth pools installed.[4,5] The fathers entered the pool as well, and often the midwife, too. He advocated use of the pool towards the end of the first stage of labour, and earlier in cases of posterior presentation and backache labour.

The first waterbirth took Michel by surprise and he stepped into the pool still wearing his socks to catch the baby. In fact, the pool was so successful in easing pain, enabling women to act instinctively, and facilitating the progress of labour, that he then installed a specially designed pool. The birth pool became the hallmark of this hospital and a symbol of his philosophy of birth.

Michel and I met at a conference on Psychoprophylaxis in Obstetrics in Rome at a time when I was living near Pithiviers, and he invited me to come and see what he was doing there. In 1977 I visited the hospital. It was not with the aim of seeing a waterbirth. Rather, it was to explore a non-obstetric mileu for birth which he had created with a group of dedicated midwives. The hospital at Pithiviers was essentially women's space, although fathers, other children and all members of the family were made welcome. As in traditional environments all over the world, birth was shaped and conducted by women.

When Odent moved to England in 1985 he brought the concept of waterbirth with him. It was enthusiastically accepted by women who were exploring alternative birth practices and the possibility of drug-free birth, and also by midwives, especially those practising independently, who saw warm water as a time-honoured and non-medical way of easing pain. Domiciliary midwives had for many years suggested that women in labour relax in a warm bath. Pools were at first used mainly in home births and midwife-run birth centres.

Women who are immersed in water in labour may want to stay in the pool for the birth. Sometimes this is an ordinary household bath. But the problem with a bath is that the sides are often narrow so that the mother cannot move easily. It may also be difficult to have the water deep enough to cover her lower torso. Instead, she is sitting in a puddle. Once birth pools were on the market there were new possibilities, above all of movement in water.

When floating in a pool, a woman in labour can move unencumbered. The water bears some of her weight and she has the sense of being in her own private world within the margins of her pool. Immersion in water enables her to move spontaneously. She squats, kneels, lies on her side, goes onto all fours, or crouches forward holding the side of the pool. Spontaneous pelvic movements that are quite difficult on land are simple in water.

She may explore gliding movements, using her arms to glide forwards and backwards during contractions or to turn from her back to one side, or from one side to the other, rolling her pelvis over as she does so. She lunges, bending one or both knees and pushing away from the side of the pool. She rolls her knees from side to side so that she is also rolling her pelvis. She rediscovers birth postures and movements that are common to traditional birth cultures all over the world.

The birth pool offered a technology that supported the special woman-to-woman relationship of the midwife and the mother. It also distanced the mother from obstetric interventions of all kinds, and from midwifery interventions such as analgesia, commanded pushing, guarding of the perineum and episiotomy. As pools came into wider use, more and more midwives observed that mothers found immersion in water comforting and that they were increasingly mobile in water.

A pool also defines the territory that is under the mother's control, in which she has autonomy, and where she can act with spontaneity, in response to the stimuli coming from her uterus and the descent and rotation of the baby's head.

In 1982, Janet Balaskas founded the Active Birth Movement. In a few years the use of water for labour and birth became one element in achieving the upright posture and pelvic mobility she advocated.[6] Pools that could be plumbed into a hospital room and portable pools started to be sold, and subsequently more birth-pool hire firms opened up (see the list of useful websites and addresses given at the end of this book).

Midwives, and some obstetricians, assisted at waterbirths in France, Switzerland, Germany and Austria and experience started to be shared internationally. In 1995 the first International Water Birth conference was held in London, organised by Janet Balaskas, Beverley Lawrence Beech, Chair of the Association for Improving the Maternity Services, and myself. Two and half thousand people attended and some of the papers were later collected in a book.[7]

At that time few British hospitals had their own pools, with the notable exception of Maidstone and the John Radcliffe in Oxford, two centres where midwifery expertise in assisting at waterbirths was developed.[8–10] However, through the 1980s and 1990s pools were installed in many National Health Service (NHS) maternity units.[11–13]

In those years too, increasing numbers of midwives in North America and Western Europe assisted at births in which women laboured, and sometimes delivered, in a birth pool. A survey into the use of water in labour and birth in England and Wales commissioned by the Department of Health revealed that, in 1993, 43% of maternity units offered a birth pool or allowed women to take in a hired pool, and all units reported that they had ordinary baths that women could use in labour. In that year, 2885 babies were born under water in Britain. In many units where there were pools, however, they were little used. Midwives lacked the confidence in assisting at waterbirths and could not develop their skills. This remains the case.

Waterbirth attracted a good deal of media attention and was the subject of scare stories based on scanty evidence.[14–16] Theses stories had the effect of sparking debate among professionals and consumer groups.[17]

The waterbirth debate

In fact, waterbirth practice still varies widely, both in Britain and around the world. Wedged on your back in a narrow bath, bouncing in a jacuzzi with high-pressure jets coming at you from all sides, sitting in a puddle of lukewarm water, perched on a pre-formed plastic elevation with legs in foot stirrups, squatting in a rocky cove of the Black Sea, clutching the sides of a huge transparent kind of goldfish-bowl, beneath bright lights, with the whole obstetric team watching, or giving birth at home, in an intimate atmosphere, with a midwife who has become a friend and your other children around you ... what exactly is waterbirth? Its all these things, and more. How do you research waterbirth when it can mean so many different things? Because there is so much cultural variety in how waterbirths are enacted, it is difficult to do a meta-analysis and to compare like with like.

Immersion in water in labour and for birth has become one of the most popular alternative birth-ways in an ever-increasing number of countries. Some UK hospitals have long lists of conditions for women who are allowed to use a pool. Yet in one Swiss hospital, which has impressive results, it is entirely up to the woman if she wants a waterbirth and, apart from the 2% of women who are transferred to a larger hospital because they deliver before the 33rd week of pregnancy, no screening is done for those using the pool.[18] In Malta, women with breech babies, twin pregnancies, those with mild hypertension, and women with previous caesarean sections are all accepted for waterbirth. No age limit is set. In an analysis of the first 1000 consecutive waterbirths in Malta, there were 89.6% spontaneous deliveries, 9.0% vacuum extractions and 1.4% caesarean sections. Of these 1000 women, 70% had an intact perineum, 24.8% had a first-degree tear, 2.9% a second-degree tear, there were no third-degree tears, and the episiotomy rate was 2.3%. Of the newborns, 98.2% had Apgar scores of 9 or more at 1 minute, 1.3% at 5 minutes, and 0.5% at 10 minutes. Only five babies were transferred to a neonatal unit and one neonatal death occurred from meconium aspiration.

Safety

The main confusion is produced by the storm of media stories about drowning babies. Oddly, obstetricians have often taken more notice of these than of research published in reputable peer-reviewed journals. This may be because the use of water in childbirth threatens obstetric territory. Waterbirth is, with few exceptions, birth attended by midwives rather than obstetricians. Few obstetricians want to wait kneeling on the floor at the side of a pool while a woman gives birth, unmanaged and undirected, in her own time and her own way.

The first birthing pool was installed in an NHS hospital in 1987. In 1992, the ground-breaking Winterton Report recommended that 'all hospitals make it their policy to make full provision for women to choose the position which they want for labour and birth, with the option of a birthing pool where this is practicable'.[19] By 1993 just under half of all hospitals provided birthing pools, while others enabled women to bring in a hired pool.

Although pools were installed, many were used infrequently. Following headlines like 'Underwater birth couple charged with manslaughter',[14] 'Waterbirth fatalities'[15] and 'Safety checks on waterbirths ordered after babies die',[16] pool rooms were turned into general storage rooms or beds were wheeled in and women told that the pool could not be used because there was no midwife on duty who had the skills required. Every time a new media scare erupted, midwives and managers became anxious and hospital protocols regarding the use of pools were tightened.

One alarm concerned the temperature of the water in the pool. It was triggered by a letter in the *Lancet* regarding the outcomes of two births in which women had been in the pool during the first stage of labour only.[20] In both cases the baby was born in poor condition and one baby died 15 hours after birth. The suggestion was made that the water may have been too hot. Fetal temperature is always at least 0.5°C greater than that of the mother. When the fetus is

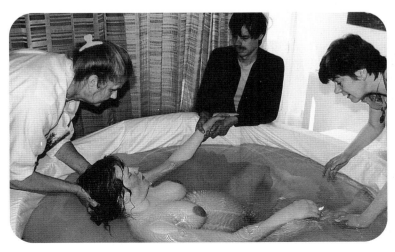

In water a woman has her own space, yet helping hands can reach her easily

overheated the basal metabolic rate and oxygen requirement increase. This could compromise an already susceptible fetus.[20] In fact, further investigation revealed that this was very unlikely to have been the cause of these babies' problems. 'The woman was not exposed to water any hotter, or for any longer, than she and all other pregnant women would experience in the course of having a bath in the normal way at home'.[21]

The main fear among those for whom waterbirth remains a mystery has always been that babies might inhale water and drown. This fear is understandable if the water fails to stimulate the vagal inspiration receptors that cause glottal closure, the so-called 'diving reflex'.[22] It may be that a baby is more likely to drink the water than breathe it in. Babies can drown when submerged, but only if they are already severely compromised and literally at their 'last gasp', or if they are kept under water following birth. This is what happened when an Austrian couple, without a midwife's help, decided that they would give their newborn the advantages of an aquatic transition to life by holding it under water for 20 minutes.

Dr Paul Johnson, a specialist in perinatal physiology, explains that fetal breathing is vigorous, intermittent (occurring about 40% of the time), and obstructed on inspiration.[22] This latter quality, which after birth will be apnoea, is essential for lung growth. Little inspiration of amniotic fluid occurs, but lung fluid, with a very low pH, is produced in the lung, comes up, and is swallowed. About 48 hours before the onset of spontaneous labour, fetal breathing stops. This may be due to the rise in prostaglandin E_2, which occurs before labour. A warm temperature also inhibits breathing, but, since the fetal temperature is higher than that of the mother, it is important that she is not overheated. Hypoxia inhibits breathing too, unless it is very severe, when gasping occurs.

It is often said that the baby has spent its fetal life in water. This is wrong. It has been in amniotic fluid. The fetus senses what is in the fluid in which it is immersed. The entrance to the larynx has more taste buds than the whole of the tongue. It is bristling with chemoreceptors and is the key in determining whether we breathe or swallow. If the baby's larynx senses water, Paul Johnson writes, breathing is inhibited and swallowing may occur, as it does in newborn lambs. Water in the larynx stimulates the diving response – apnoea, swallowing, arousal, bradycardia and hypertension, and blood flow is distributed to the brain, heart and adrenal glands. Many medical drugs block the diving response. The fetus knows its own environmental and body fluids and responds differently to foreign fluids. As can be observed in many videos of waterbirth, a baby born under warm water after spontaneous onset of labour, undrugged, with its cord intact, and not asphyxiated, is inhibited from breathing until it surfaces into cooler air.[22]

Paediatricians and managers often raised the issue of infection. In fact one London teaching hospital required all women using a pool to take a test for the human immunodeficiency virus (HIV) first. A resulting enquiry by the Expert Advisory Group on AIDS of the Department of Health concluded that 'There is no evidence that HIV is any more likely to be transmitted from mother to baby in a birthing pool than during birth elsewhere'. Testing of patients should not be used as a substitute for adequate protection of health. It is the responsibility of caregivers at all times to prevent contact with potentially infective blood, body fluids or, in this case, contaminated water. There were no circumstances where it is acceptable to test expectant mothers for HIV purely as a condition of using birthing pools.[23] Research showed that babies born in water were no more likely to have infections than those born conventionally. It is accepted good practice to clean pools with chlorine-releasing agents, which are effective against HIV and hepatitis B and C.

Following concerns about safety, a major paediatric epidemiological study, based on the Institute of Child Health in London, compared outcomes for 4032 babies born in water in England and Wales with those of all babies born in air over the same 2-year period.[24] Fifteen hundred paediatricians reported deaths and admissions to special care following water immersion in labour and/or at birth each month from April 1994 to April 1996. Perinatal mortality for babies born in water was 1.2 per 1000 live births. Perinatal mortality in babies of women at low risk of complications who delivered conventionally ranges from 0.8 to 4.6 per 1000 births in different parts of Britain. Of five perinatal deaths among the babies born in water, two were stillborn, one after a concealed pregnancy with no prenatal care, born unattended at home, and the was other diagnosed as a stillbirth before the mother entered the water. The three postpartum deaths indicated abnormal physiological findings, but no deaths could be directly attributed to waterbirth. Admissions to special care for babies of low-risk primiparous women generally were significantly higher for those born in air than for those born in water. In Scottish hospitals the numbers ranged from 8.4 per 1000 for babies born in water to 64 per 1000 for normal women with spontaneous vaginal deliveries.

In five cases the umbilical cord of babies born in water snapped, which is not an emergency for a skilled midwife. In fact, it is not known how often this occurs with land births. But one result of this study is that midwives assisting at waterbirth are now advised to avoid traction on the cord and to bring the baby up into the mother's arms slowly.

There is also the fear of pneumonia associated with waterbirth. Nguyen[25] described four babies who were admitted to hospital with respiratory difficulties after waterbirth, but no details of the births were available, so it is impossible to conclude that waterbirth was the cause of their problems.

Gilbert[26] subsequently wrote a letter on waterbirth in *Pediatrics* in which she referred to 'several reports of death attributable to drowning resulting from poorly managed waterbirth'. These are the ones described by Zimmerman,[27] some of which were recorded after unsubstantiated reports in a waterbirth workshop in Switzerland. One of these deaths was in France. The baby was born with intact membranes in an unattended birth and the parents did not rupture

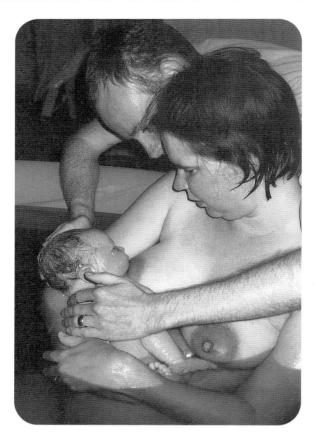

A baby is lifted out of the water and straight to the mother's breast – a gentle transition to life

them. They only realised the baby was not alive after about an hour. Another is the birth in Austria to which I have already referred, when the parents left the baby submerged for 20 minutes.[21]

Over and above the effects of waterbirth on babies, a concern often raised is that midwives may hurt their backs through stretching and lifting a woman in a pool. Some hospitals installed hoists, rather like mini industrial cranes, projecting over the pool to raise the mother if she collapsed. But, because women using pools have usually not received opioids or other analgesics, it has become obvious that women are very unlikely to lose consciousness, and no case of this has been reported. Moreover, once midwives gain experience with pool births, they realise that they rarely need to guard the perineum, feel for the nuchal cord or assist restitution of the baby's head, and that, because these manoeuvres can theoretically stimulate premature breathing, such interventions are best avoided.

There is strong evidence from observational studies that immersion in water relieves pain and that women who are in a pool are less likely to have drugs for pain relief.[18, 28–33] In the rather stilted language of research studies, waterbirth 'increases maternal satisfaction'.[34] Randomised controlled trials of immersion in water during labour, but not giving birth under water, also show that women need fewer pain-killing drugs.[35, 36] One randomised controlled trial showed that babies were less likely to be posterior when the mother laboured in water.[37]

The birth pool is now on the way to being considered a standard birth option for low-risk women, not an alternative form of care. Moreover, research proposals are being considered to explore the possibilities of the use of a pool in births where there are known risk factors. With new monitors that can be used under water and allow the mother freedom to move, women experiencing (that dreadful term) a 'trial of scar' may benefit from birth pools. Immersion in water may also be helpful in labours where it has been taken for granted that high-tech treatment is the obvious way. We know that being able to relax in warm water in a peaceful setting, with lights dimmed and no intrusive sounds, hurried movements or other interventions, reduces blood pressure. So, a birth pool might become a treatment for hypertension.

It may help when the cervix is slow to dilate, too. A small study to evaluate labour during the first stage in multiparous women with dystocia revealed that, compared with amniotomy and intravenous oxytocin, women who used a birth pool had fewer epidurals. They were also less likely to need uterine stimulation or any kind of obstetric intervention. Using a birth pool did not affect the caesarean rate.[38] The author suggests that immersion in water is not only an alternative way of managing pain, but also helps when labour is slow, and is beneficial because it reduces intervention.

Waterbirth is, almost without exception, to do with the midwife's conduct of labour, and obstetricians are rarely involved. Obstetricians who attend waterbirths learn new ways of assisting at birth, acquiring midwifery skills as they adapt to waterbirths. Some have witnessed births without any intervention for the first time, and without procedures that are usually accepted as innocuous, such as artificial rupture of the membranes, drugs for pain relief, manipulative delivery of the baby's head, and routine suction of the newborn. A Professor of Obstetrics told me he had just seen a waterbirth in his hospital. 'It was amazing!' he said. 'The baby just sort of floated out!'

One problem, however, is that many midwives have limited opportunity to develop the skills they need to assist at waterbirths with confidence. The Midwives' Rules of Practice[39] state that when midwives use 'complementary and alternative therapies ... it is essential that practice in these respects, as in all others, is based upon sound principles and upon all available knowledge and skill'. An experienced waterbirth midwife and researcher, Ethel Burns, has a programme of study days for midwives in hospitals that have pools, or are considering installing pools. Drawing on the available evidence, Ethel Burns and I have developed *Midwifery Guidelines for the use of Water in Labour*.[40]

All forms of care in childbirth need to be rigorously evaluated. This includes practices often accepted because they are customary. Many such practices – enemas and perineal shaving, immobilisation and the supine position for labour and delivery, the use of lithotomy stirrups, commanded pushing and prolonged breath-holding, and routine episiotomy – have been questioned only in the last 25 years. The introduction of new technologies, methods of management and forms of pain relief require equally rigorous analysis. It is not only immersion in hot water that might cause fever in the baby. Epidural anaesthesia, for example, produces pyrexia in both mother and baby.[41] Yet little concern has been expressed about this side-effect of epidurals.

Women who give birth in water feel more in control[42] and are more likely to look back on the experience happily than those who give birth on land – in the same hospital, with the same caregivers, and provided with other options that enable them to be upright.[18]

Some midwives are expert in deflecting women from labouring or giving birth in water, either because they themselves are fearful or sometimes because they cannot be bothered. The following are some of the reasons that midwives give as to why a woman cannot use the birth pool:

- We don't have a midwife trained in waterbirth.
- Your blood pressure is slightly raised.
- It hasn't been cleaned yet.
- I'm going off duty.
- Your notes say that your last baby was born pre-term.
- The room isn't free. (Hidden agenda here: the Senior House Officer is sleeping there.)
- The room isn't free. (Hidden agenda here: we're using it as a store room.)
- Your notes say that you had a caesarean section the time before last.
- It's a long way up the hall from the midwives' station.
- The hoist hasn't been installed yet.
- We couldn't monitor the baby if you were in the pool.
- Your notes say that you had an episiotomy last time.
- You may need a caesarean section.
- We can't find the thermometer.
- I have a bad back.
- Something has gone wrong with the pool.
- I don't do waterbirths.
- Someone else is in it (a week ago).

When such ploys are used, the choice of waterbirth is spurious. The option is presented to make women think that there are alternatives to routine, regimented care and to keep them quiet. This is not just a matter of individual staff being dishonest or deceitful. It is an expression of the ways in which those in power use their position to manipulate women in childbirth and keep the system running as *they* want it, not as those at the receiving end of care would like it. As a midwife in the Informed Choice study said, 'Informed choice is really about women using their initiative to find out what is not available, rather than what is'.[43]

References

1.   Kitzinger S 2000 Rediscovering birth. London: Little Brown, pp 195–196
2.   Kitzinger S 1989 Labouring in a Soviet time warp. The Independent, 6 June 1989
3.   LeBoyer F 1977 Birth without violence. London: Fontana

4. Odent M 1983 Birth under water. Lancet ii:1376–1377

5. Odent M 1990 Water and sexuality. London: Penguin

6. Balaskas J 1988 Waterbirth. New Generation 7(2):5–6

7. Beech BL 1996 Water birth unplugged. Hale: Books for Midwives

8. Garland D, Jones K 1997 Waterbirth: updating the evidence. British Journal of Midwifery 5(6)

9. Garland D 1995 Waterbirth – an attitude to care. Hale: Books for Midwives

10. Burns E, Greenish K 1993 Pooling information. Nursing Times 89(8):47–49

11. Kitzinger S 1991 Letter from England. Birth 18(3)

12. Alderdice F, Renfrew M, Marchant S, et al 1995 Labour and birth in water in England and Wales. BMJ 310(6983):837

13. Brown L 1998 The tide has turned: audit of water birth. British Journal of Midwifery 6(4)

14. Underwater birth couple charged with manslaughter. Daily Telegraph, 29 September 1990

15. Water birth fatalities. The Independent, 16 October 1993

16. Safety checks on water births ordered after babies die. The Daily Telegraph, 16 October 1993

17. Page L, Kitzinger S 1995 A midwifery perspective on the use of water in labour and birth. Maternal and Child Health, 22 January 1995

18. Geissbühler V, Eberhard J 2000 Waterbirths: a comparative study. Fetal Diagnosis and Therapy 15(5):291–300

19. House of Commons Health Committee 1992 Report on maternity services 1992. Second report, vol 11, p xcviii. London: HMSO

20. Rosevear SK, Fox R, Marlow N, et al 1993 Birthing pools and the fetus [letter]. Lancet 342(8878):1048–1049

21. Rosser J 1994 Is waterbirth safe? The facts behind the controversy. MIDIRS Midwifery Digest 4(1):4–6

22. Johnson P 1996 Birth under water – to breathe or not to breathe. British Journal of Obstetrics and Gynaecology 103(3):202–203

23. Metters JS 1996 Letter from Deputy Chief Medical Officer, Department of Health to Dr Peter Brocklehurst, Director, National Perinatal Epidemiology Unit, Oxford. 15 May

24. Gilbert RE, Tookey PA 1999 Perinatal morality and morbidity among babies delivered in water: surveillance study and postal survey. BMJ 319(7208):483–487

25. Nguyen S, Kuschel C, Teele R, et al 2002 Water birth – a near-drowning experience. Pediatrics 110(2):411–413

26. Gilbert R 2002 Water birth – a near drowning experience [letter]. Pediatrics 110(2 Pt 1):409

27. Zimmermann R, Huch A, Huch R 1993 Water birth – is it safe? Journal of Perinatal Medicine 21(1):5–11

28. Garland D, Jones K 1994 Waterbirth: 'first-stage' immersion or non-immersion? British Journal of Midwifery 2:113–19

29. Burke E, Kilfoyle A 1995 A comparative study: waterbirth and bedbirth. Midwives 108:327

30. Eldering G 1995 Water birth – a possible mode of delivery? In: Beech BAL (ed) Water birth unplugged. Proceedings of the First International Water Birth Conference. Hale: Books for Midwives Press

31. Burns E, Lloyd A 2001 Waterbirth. MIDIRS Midwifery Digest 11(3 Suppl 2)

32. Otigbah CM, Dhanjal MK, Harmsworth G, et al 2000 A retrospective comparison of water births and conventional vaginal deliveries. European Journal of Obstetrics, Gynecology and Reproductive Biology 91(1):15–20

33. Moneta J, Okninska A, Wielgos M, et al 2001 The influence of water immersion on the course of labor [in Polish]. Ginekologika Politica 72(12):1031–1036

34. Cluett ER, Nikodem VC, McCandlish RE, Burns EE 2004 Immersion in water in pregnancy, labour and birth. Cochrane Database Systematic Review 2:CD000111

35. Rush J, Burlock S, Lambert K, et al 1996 The effects of whirlpool baths in labor: a randomized, controlled trial. Birth 23(3):136–143

36. Cammu H, Clasen K, Van Wettere L, et al 1994 'To bathe or not to bathe' during the first stage of labor. Acta Obstetrica et Gynecologica Scandinavica 73(6):468–472

37. Ohlsson G, Buchhave P, Leandersson U, et al 2001 Warm tub bathing during labor: maternal and neonatal effects. Acta Obstetrica et Gynecologica Scandinavica 80(4):311–314

38. Cluett ER, Pickering RM, Geeliffe K, et al 2004 Randomised controlled trial of labouring in water compared with standard of augmentation for management of dystocia in first stage of labour. BMJ 328(7435):314

39. UKCC 1998 Midwives' rules of practice. London: UKCC, p 34. Updated – midwives rules and standards. London: Nursing & Midwifery Council, 2004. Available at: http://www.nmc-uk.org (accessed November 2004)

40. Burns E, Kitzinger S 2000 Midwifery guidelines for the use of water in labour. Oxford: Brookes University. Order form available at: http://www.sheilakitzinger.com\waterbirth.htm. Workshop information available from Ethel Burns at: eburns@brookes.ac.uk

41. Lieberman E, Lang J, Richardson DK, et al 2000 Intrapartum maternal fever and neonatal outcome. Pediatrics 105:8–13

42. Hall SM, Holloway IM 1998 Staying in control: women's experiences of labour in water. Midwifery 14(1):30–36

43. Stapleton H 2004 Is there a difference between a free gift and a planned purchase? The use of evidence-based leaflets in maternity care. In: Kirkham M (ed) Informed choice in maternity care. New York: Palgrave MacMillan, p 100

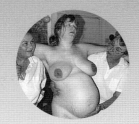

14
Birth dance

Birth is movement

To an observer it may be almost imperceptible – a ripple of movement down the spine as the uterus contracts, the fundus hardens and tilts forward, the baby's head is pressed down, and the woman takes more pronounced audible breaths. Yet it is always there. Perhaps she swings her legs to one side, bends her knees, grips with her feet, lifts her buttocks as she presses down with the palms of her hands. Perhaps she rocks her pelvis forward and back, circles in long, slow swoops, or tilts her pelvis, stretching along one side, in response to the heavy pressure she feels as her whole abdomen becomes hard and feels as if it swells up like a great wave and the baby descends even deeper. She leans forward, curves her lower back or arches it, crouches or kneels. Perhaps she stands and lunges.

With each contraction there is breathing and movement. In every country where I have been with women in childbirth I have seen them either moving freely or struggling to move. There was no need for them to be taught or coached in the birth dance. All they needed was to be free to do it.

Only if a woman is numbed from the waist down does this spontaneous movement cease. Then she is in an anaesthetic straitjacket. The labour must proceed without her. She can no longer dance. It comes as no surprise that this increases the chance of delivery needing to be assisted with forceps or ventouse and makes it more likely that the baby will have to be extracted by caesarean section.

The Cochrane Database includes a review of positions in the second stage of labour, but not positions that women have been free to choose themselves, nor how these may vary at different phases of the birth process and with babies presenting differently, nor in varied kinds of labour (for example, slow, rapid or backache labour), because comparative studies at this level do not exist.

Nor does the Cochrane Database provide information about *movement*, either movements suggested by the caregiver or those chosen by the mother. We cannot learn much from the Cochrane negative finding that upright positions are not harmful, although there may be increased blood loss – the 'may' is important because upright positions might possibly allow for more accurate measurement – so women should be helped to choose the positions they prefer.[1] Perhaps that research has missed the point. It may not be static positions that are most helpful, but *movement between positions.*

Postures for delivery in traditional cultures have been recorded since Dr George Engelmann and a medical student, Robert Felkin, described them in North American native cultures and African tribes in the 19th century.[2] Although information about how women move in labour has been reported incidentally, pelvic mobility and ways of encouraging this by providing physical support can be observed all over the world. The result is movement that constitutes, in effect, a birth dance. This is in stark contrast to the immobility imposed on women in a technocratic birth culture, where they are expected to lie on a bed or delivery table, harpooned to an intravenous drip and electronic equipment, and are told to keep still so as not to interfere with the fetal monitor. It is a culture where pain-killing drugs also reduce the mother's awareness and may even paralyse every part of her body beneath her breasts.

Before the delivery table was invented women were often upright or semi-upright as they moved. They stood, squatted, or half-leant, half-squatted, grasping stakes set in the ground or the central house pole. Or they held a rope or long strip of cloth suspended from a beam, and knotted at the lower end, and swung on it with each contraction. Often another woman, or sometimes the father of the baby, held the mother from behind and moved with her. A further variation was when she stood, a woman at either side, arms around her, who moved in synchrony with her. Birth then became a dance with two partners.

A combination of having a bar or pole to grasp and walking around in between contractions was common. In Montana, the Flathead woman grasped a horizontal bar fixed between two upright posts so that she was able to rock her pelvis, and gave birth supported by another woman on a skin spread with soft bison wool. In Central Africa the Banyoro woman alternately grasped a stick driven into the ground and walked in a circle round it.

Japanese women traditionally adopted many different positions for the second stage. The mother held on to a rope hanging from the ceiling, and moved between half-sitting and standing. She might kneel leaning against a pile of straw bundles and a quilt, or sit leaning back with the midwife or her husband holding her pelvis from behind, or she might crouch forward over a bed of rice, or kneel with her back supported by futons. There are myths that one empress gave birth to twins while leaning against a mortar, and that another delivered her son while holding on to a branch of the pagoda tree at a shrine.[3]

When a woman laboured out of doors, as she might in the New Guinea forest or in the African bush, she often walked around and grasped the trunk or branch of a tree as each contraction came. Today women are rediscovering the advantages of pelvic movement during labour and, rather than using special equipment for support, hold onto furniture, a partner or, if they give birth at home, even a tree in the garden.

Among some native North Americans it was the practice to erect a palisade of branches with stakes pushed into the ground at measured intervals, forming a path leading to an inner sanctum. The woman walked from stake to stake as her labour progressed. It provided visible evidence of the advance of labour, and when she reached the second stage at last she reached the inner space where she was to give birth.

A Hopi woman squatted or knelt on a sheepskin in a corner of the birth room, walking between contractions. Bedouin Arab girls learn pelvic movements for sex and birth in the ceremonies that herald adulthood. This is the origin of the North African belly dance. It is slow and languorous, quite different from the rapid gyrations and jerks of night club belly dancing.

Kneeling was often made easier by using birth stones or bricks. In Egypt women knelt on two birth stones. In the King James Bible this was translated as 'stools': 'And the King of Egypt spoke to the Hebrew midwives ... and he said "when ye do the office of midwife to the Hebrew women and seat them upon the stools"'. This was a loose rendering of an Egyptian word that meant 'a pair of stones'. Kneeling on them, a woman could rock back and forth.

An alternative was to sit between the thighs of another woman. Rachel says of the labour of her maidservant, Bilha, 'She shall bear upon my knees that I may also have children by her'.

We have seen already in Chapter 3 that birth stools were used widely in Europe in the past. Midwives carried their own stools with them till well into the 19th century. They were a vital part of their equipment. They are mentioned in the very first obstetric textbook, written in the 2nd century AD, and were popular throughout North Africa and Europe. When the mother sat on a stool women helpers offered their own bodies to support her from behind. Only later were backs constructed for these stools. At first they were sloped so that the woman could move her pelvis, but by the 16th century in Germany the stools had evolved into birth chairs, and it was the midwife who sat on a stool in front of the woman.

The more elaborate birth chairs became, the harder they were to transport, and the more difficult it was for the woman to move. She was more or less upright, but fixed in one position, with intricate carving pressing against her neck and arms. In the 13th century Haggabbah of Sarejevo, miniature paintings show the birth of Rebecca's twins with the mother sitting on a birth stool and the midwife kneeling at her feet. By the 16th century German illustrations depict women sitting on elaborate birth chairs, with the midwife either on a stool or kneeling at their feet, always with other women attending. In the 19th century the Prussian consul in Jerusalem wrote that peasant women gave birth on stones, but wealthier women used birth chairs.

In 2002, American archaeologists discovered some Ancient Egyptian birth bricks in a 3700-year-old palace. They excavated one elaborately decorated and colourful birth brick that shows a mother with her newborn, attended on either side by helping women and by Hathor, the Cow Goddess of birth and motherhood.

Birth bricks are still used by women in India. Nowadays they are ordinary builders' bricks, which they even take into hospital with them.

Unaccustomed as we are to hammocks, except to lie in the garden, it may seem that they curtail mobility, and that all you can do with a hammock is to collapse in it. But in South America babies are conceived, cradled and born in hammocks. Hammocks are cheap, familiar, flexible, washable, biodegradable, and can be adapted to different activities. In the Amazon, tribal women give birth in a closely woven cotton hammock into which a large hole has been cut, and the baby drops through it onto warm, soft ashes or into a water-filled canoe. In Mexico and Guatemala a woman gives birth in her old hammock, with a new hammock hanging above it on which she pulls during contractions. After the birth the old hammock is discarded and she and the baby move into the new one.

This practice can be adapted easily to contemporary hospital practice. A hammock or cloth sling attached to a strong hook in the ceiling enables a woman to stand, squat or kneel leaning into it and to use gravity to help her bear down. It should be fixed so that it can be raised or lowered, depending on how she wishes to use it.[4]

The death of the dance

In the 20th century, as European and American obstetrics spread to South America, Africa and beyond, medicalised birth was superimposed on traditional cultures, and caregivers went to great lengths to ensure that women obeyed instructions and complied with 'modern' and 'scientific' methods. With the invention of the delivery table women were prevented from moving and were fixed to a metal slab. The positions imposed on them were designed to make the uterus and vulva easily accessible to the obstetrician so that he could employ various manoeuvres – each of which was labelled in the textbooks with the name of the obstetrician who originally devised it.

An English medical student who worked in Algeria in the 1970s describes an event in the hospital delivery room:

> It's her eighth delivery, and her first in hospital … She's been in labour all night. Her cervix is fully open and the baby's head is where it should be,

ready to come down. But something's wrong. Her contractions are short and weak. She doesn't seem to have her heart in the whole business. Djamila [the midwife] *wags a finger and threatens the woman in French, which she doesn't understand: 'If you're not careful, Dr Kostov will come and give you a big spanking'. She gets up on the bed and kneels beside the woman, pressing down on her belly with both hands, arms stiff and straight, trying to push the baby out. To no avail. We go out on to the landing to rest.*

We come back to find the woman squatting on the floor, holding herself upright by the bedpost. Fatma the Kabyl cleaner screams. Djamila spits Arab war-cries. They shoo the woman back on to the bed. Djamila won't hear of delivering her on the floor. She's scandalised. She's never seen it done, but she knows there must be a good reason against it. Women deliver on their backs, all else is primitive.

... Djamila's wounded, and she falls on to the chair in the corner. She'll have nothing more to do with the woman, who's telling Fatma that she won't go anywhere else but on the floor. She always squatted before, and that's what she's going to do now. If they won't let her, she's going to sleep. She stretches out her legs, throws down her robe and closes her eyes.[5]

During field work in Moscow in the 1970s I witnessed how, after the ritual complete shave and enema, the woman was put on a narrow, hard, high bed to 'get on with it'. She lay alone, biting her lips, moaning quietly, or writhing in silent agony. When it was judged time for the baby to be born she was wheeled to the delivery room, had to climb on a table, lie flat on her back, and push as hard and as often as she could. A hurried, violent delivery was conducted by an obstetrician, who entered the room solely for this purpose and then left. This is how the second stage is managed in hospitals all over the world where midwifery is not strong, practice is not evidence-based, and the primary concern of caregivers is to tether the mother in a position for convenient obstetric manoeuvres and deliver the baby as fast as possible.

References

1. Gupta JK, Nicodem VC 2000 Women's position during second stage of labour. Cochrane Database Systematic Review 2:CD002006. Update in: Cochrane Database Systematic Review 2004;1:CD002006

2. Kitzinger S 2000 Rediscovering birth. London: Little Brown, pp 177–191

3. Ritsuko T (ed) 1990 Childbirth in Japan. Tokyo: Birth International

4. Kitzinger S 2003 The new pregnancy and childbirth. London: Dorling Kindersley, pp 218–19

5. Young I 1974 The private life of Islam. London: Allen Lane, pp 19–20

15
What's happening to midwives?

The whole system of maternity care in Britain is based on midwifery. Because obstetricians are specialists in pathology, without midwives care in childbirth would collapse, and most women would have to give birth attended only by family and friends.

Throughout western European countries midwives are the main caregivers. What doctors learn about normal birth they acquire largely from midwives. On the whole, women do not need obstetricians, but there is no question that they need midwives.

Midwifery philosophy is based on acknowledging and supporting natural processes, intervening only when necessary, and advocating for women and their families. 'The underlying framework of the midwifery model is the understanding and value of connection; the understanding of relatedness of the body and mind, mother and baby, midwife and woman, and woman and her social context'.[1]

Wherever autonomous midwifery exists and midwives can work as colleagues with obstetricians, and are not their handmaidens, perinatal mortality rates are the lowest in the world. This is the case in the Scandinavian countries, The Netherlands and New Zealand, where one-third of births take place at home. Midwives are qualified to provide total care in pregnancy, birth and afterwards. In spite of this, they have had little influence on formulating public health policies, and institutions representing obstetricians speak with a louder and more authoritative voice. In Germany and Italy, maternity clinics are similar to the US model. When I observed births in hospitals in northern Italy, for example, I witnessed women waiting to give birth until the obstetrician put in an appearance. They were ordered not to push, however much they wanted to.

Midwives were not supposed to deliver, except in an emergency. The obstetrician entered, performed an episiotomy, and delivered, often employing fundal pressure and using a manoeuvre that entails sticking a finger in the woman's anus and rapidly forcing the baby's chin up over the perineum (which is why the episiotomy was essential).

In eastern Europe, Communism introduced a totalitarian and highly bureaucratic medical control of childbirth. It is still the norm. Zuzana Stromerova, of the Czech Association of Midwives, says: 'Under the Communist regime midwives were a small body of professionals who had little power and had to do as they were told'.[2] There is no midwifery legislation and no laws referring to midwifery in the Czech Republic. Midwives are not recognised legally as an autonomous profession and are called 'women's nurses', although a law passed by Parliament in 2004 at last gives midwives new professional recognition. Zuzana went on to say that doctors 'view a normal birth as a potential crisis, not a normal event in life, and it is doctors who are considered the "experts". Hospitals are not paid by health insurance companies unless there is a signature from the doctor on duty or chief doctor'. So an independent midwife, if it were possible for her to exist, would get paid nothing. Birth is the responsibility of obstetricians. Out-of-hospital births are forbidden by law, and a midwife can be punished for helping a women have a planned home birth, as can the mother too.

A World Health Organisation (WHO) report on midwifery in central and eastern European countries states:

> Doctors are the lead professionals in birth ... Midwives hold the position of doctor's assistant and are often not advocates of women. Home birth is neither attended by midwives nor supported ... Midwives provide care immediately following the birth but not in the postnatal period...Midwifery practise is not based on the latest evidence and research ... Legislation states that 'Midwives work under the authority/direction of a doctor'. There is no register for practising midwives ... Midwives have little influence in the setting of national policies ... No local structures exist which monitor standards of midwifery practice.[3]

Commenting on midwifery education, the WHO report[3] observes that up to 65% of time is spent on theory and never more than 40% on practice: 'There are no midwifery training establishments. There are no nursing establishments affiliated with institutes of higher education'.

The situation is particularly bad in Hungary. Maternal and child health nurses, not midwives, are the primary carers of pregnant women. Midwives work under the supervision of doctors and, according to WHO, although midwifery practice is claimed to be evidence-based, it 'is dependent on the physician's practice and philosophy of the institution'.[4] Home births are banned. The Board of Hungarian Obstetricians and Gynaecologists has issued two statements about home birth: 'Pregnancy is a biological process that has several special pathophysiological features even in "normal" cases' and 'Pregnant women must not endanger the health or life of their fetuses/new-born babies by rejecting birth in a clinic/hospital'.

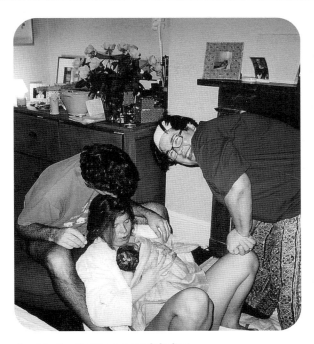

A midwife shares a couple's joy

'The restoration of home births would, even after significant investments, endanger the safety of child-births, and put the health and lives of mothers and new-born babies at risk'.[4] Section 17(2)(a) of the Health Care Act proclaims that 'pregnant women do not have the right to autonomously decide in this issue, and thus cannot reject maternity treatment in hospital'. and 'The outstanding results of Hungary's obstetrics in reducing perinatal mortality have always been accreditable to institutional births'.

'Women about to give birth need the constant availability of emergency services'.[5] The Health Care Act rules that 'a pregnant woman must not reject life-saving or life-maintaining intervention. Pregnancy is not among the exceptional situations when a patient is legally allowed to reject health-care provisions'. That includes delivery in hospital and compliance with any obstetric interventions that are considered necessary by the professionals in charge.

Ten new members joined the European Union (EU) in 2004, including these eastern European nations. They are required to change their maternity care systems to meet the EU standard and will have to give midwives professional and autonomous status, although they are allowed 2 years in which to make these adjustments. It is a huge challenge. As I write (2004), midwives in Eire which joined the EU in 1973, still have no supportive legislation and have been waiting for recognition for 6 years.

Meanwhile, there is a new restlessness among midwives in the UK, with lively debate about how to promote normal childbirth, really listen to women, and work with those who want to avoid obstetric interventions and high-tech management. Midwifery is also being examined in terms of the needs of a society in which deprivation starts, for many people, at birth. In 2004, the UK Government published a National Service Framework for children, young people and the maternity services, and midwives are in the forefront of initiatives to identify how they can serve the most vulnerable in our society. Sure Start projects have begun to address drug and alcohol addiction in pregnancy, and the needs of teenage pregnant women, ethnic minority families and travellers. More options for home birth are opening up, together with birthing units run by midwives. Meryl Thomas, Vice President of the Royal College of Midwives, says: 'There is evidence that women wish to have, and improved outcomes are more assured by, one-to-one care by a midwife for a woman throughout labour'.[6, 7] 'There is also a significant number of women who would like to have a non-interventionist, normal childbirth experience and the option to give birth in a midwifery-led environment, or in a purpose designed birthing centre'.[6, 8] She stresses that midwifery is an autonomous profession and that 'capitulation to the views of other professionals is not appropriate, whereas reasoned argument is'.

On the other hand, British midwives are leaving midwifery in droves. There are 43,590 registered midwives, of whom 32,190 are practising (figures for 31 March 2003). So 11,400 qualified midwives are not practising. For some this is because they simply wanted a midwifery qualification in order to get a senior post as a healthcare professional. The midwife shortage is often discussed by policy-makers as if it were solely a matter of low pay and working conditions that are incompatible with family life. Both of these may be true. But there is more to it. Many are dissatisfied because they did not go into midwifery to spend their time filling in forms, manipulating machinery, and having to switch their attention between three or four women in labour at the same time, leaving them supervised only by continuous electronic fetal monitors and rendered compliant with epidurals. They entered midwifery to give woman-to-woman care. Mothers often do not receive this quality of care, and midwives are denied the opportunity to give it.

There is evidence that midwives find that their work is most satisfying when there is continuity.[9] Everyone agrees that continuity is a good thing in the health services. But the concept needs to be deconstructed. It does not just mean that services are integrated at management level or that systems such as care pathways and care management are adopted. It has to do with personal *experience*. 'For continuity to exist, care must be experienced by individuals as connected and coherent ... and the perception that different providers agree on the management plan, and that a provider who knows them will care for them in the future'.[10]

A multidisciplinary study by researchers working in Canada, England and the USA defined three types of continuity:

- *informational continuity* – the use of information of past events and personal circumstances 'to make current care appropriate for each individual'
- *management continuity* – 'a consistent and coherent approach to ... management ... that is responsive to a patient's changing needs'
- *relational continuity* – 'an ongoing therapeutic relationship between a patient and one or more providers'.

It is this relational continuity that is important in maternity care for both childbearing women and midwives.[11] Continuity exists for a midwife when care is not fragmented, is given over time, and there is a focus on individual women.

Inflexibility: by design or default?

Continuity is not just a matter of conveying information accurately, or of conforming to thin guidelines or developing joint policies. It is, at best, continuity of *relationships*. This is difficult to ensure when a large team has to share responsibility for a woman's care, especially when midwives are overworked and pressed for time. They have to pass on case details like a baton being handed between marathon runners. The tendency is for the recorded data, rather than the human being, to be the focus of information and interest.[10] For an idealistic midwife this is highly stressful, and there is inherent conflict between professionalism and personal caring.

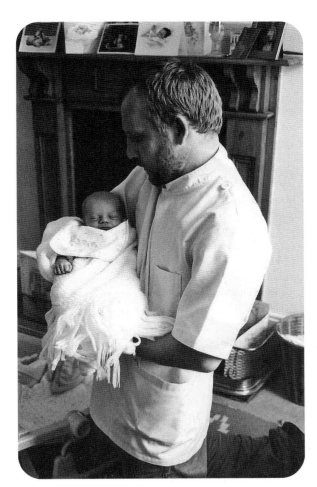

Midwife Paul Beland – dismissed for attending a home birth in 2004 (see p. 110)

Team midwifery, although ostensibly designed to meet patients' needs, in fact bolsters midwives' support from a professional group that reinforces their status and the established belief system, but undermines their relationship with individual women. It is taken for granted that when mothers are seen as difficult or deviant the midwife's first allegiance should be to the team. However much an individual midwife may want to give a woman individual care,

145

acknowledge her autonomy, and her right to give birth in the way she wants, it is easiest to adapt to the dominant ethos of the team. The midwife's professional future may depend on it.

An alternative to teams is caseload or one-to-one midwifery, in which a midwife, working with a partner, cares for a woman through pregnancy, birth and the post-partum period. Professor Lesley Page writes that, for midwives, 'There is a world of difference between being with childbearing women through the entire journey of pregnancy and birth, and providing random and fragmented care to a number of different women'.[12]

A named midwife cares for 40 women a year in a small geographical area, on her personal caseload. She plans around four births a month. In one such system, 92% of women in labour were attended by a known midwife, 75% by the named midwife, and 17% by the named midwife's partner.[13] As Lesley Page points out: 'In one-to-one practice, one midwife and her partner are on call for eight births per month, compared with team midwifery where, with a team caseload of 240 births per year, team midwives are on call for 20 births per month. In addition, communications are simpler, and it is not as complicated to ensure that the woman knows both of the midwives. If, however, a "team" of six undertakes to do a 1 in 6 rota, the midwife is far more likely to be called out on her night on call, is more likely to have a number of women in labour at once and has a higher chance of being called for women she does not know well or even at all'.

But reorganisation of working arrangements, although giving the midwife more autonomy and responsibility, is unlikely by itself to put the heart back into midwifery. National statistics prepared by the UK Government Statistical Service reveal that births conducted by midwives fell from 76% in 1989/90 to 65% in 2001/02. The percentage of women who gave birth 'without intervention' (i.e. no induction, spinal, epidural, or general anaesthesia, and no instrumental delivery or caesarean section) fell from 56% in 1991/92 to 45% in 2001/02, and the proportion of hospital deliveries that occurred spontaneously fell from 78% in 1989 to 67% in 2001/02. That is, in each case, a drop of 11%.[14]

Midwives find themselves in stressful situations in which they are overworked, understaffed and expected to undertake high-tech interventions. The response of management has been to instruct midwives working in the community – those who attend home births, for example – to come into the delivery suite to help out, and also to employ 'bank' midwives to fill in.

Research into 'near misses' and 'adverse events' – accidents waiting to happen – in seven maternity units in the north-west of England revealed that everywhere there were too few midwives to take responsibility for high-risk practices, including the administration of drugs to induce labour and to stimulate labour once labour had started (rates ranged from 25% to 59%) and epidural anaesthesia (rates ranged from 11% to 35%), which continued in spite of midwife shortages.[15] It turned out that these high-risk practices occurred most often in units with the most severe staff shortages. The authors of this study state: 'Analysis of the previously identified 3 months' near misses revealed that an alarming percentage of them (78–95%) involved the use of oxytocin for induction or acceleration, epidural blockades, or both'.

It also emerged that midwives were frequently switched from clinical work to clerical duties. They were so pressed for time that they could not acquire training or update their skills in cardiotocography or managing emergencies, and so their confidence was eroded. There was a poor skill mix on the labour ward, associated with composition of teams in which relatively inexperienced midwives often had no skilled midwives working alongside them from whom they could learn. The conclusion arrived at was rather odd: 'Midwives are fundamental components in the system of intrapartum care', referring to them as if they were cogs in a machine.[15]

The researchers failed to discuss the effects of the emphasis on high-risk practices in depriving midwives of the opportunity to learn how to support normal labour. Labour-management policies downgrade the skills of keeping birth normal, concentrating instead on interventionist practices that suck midwives away from attending women who otherwise might have physiological rather than medicalised or surgical births.

These interventionist practices are often not acknowledged, because they are not seen. Many midwifery interventions have a positive effect. There are many more that can be harmful. Tricia Anderson suggests that they can be categorised at three levels.[16] Her analysis is given in Tables 15.1 and 15.2. She writes: 'When we have a vocabulary of basic midwifery interventions, we can then start to have a dialogue about when it might be appropriate to move from a 1st level intervention, to a 2nd or 3rd level one'. She is not for one moment suggesting complete inaction. 'There is an inherent and very real danger in a newly qualified midwife who thinks all she has to do is sit on a sofa and knit! I feel a slight ripple of concern when midwives say they are *always* "hands off" the perineum or they *never* use directed pushing, for example'. A midwife needs to be relaxed, but alert and watchful, even when she may seem to be doing nothing.

With increasing dependence on technology and more obstetric intervention, midwifery skills are eroded. At the same time, midwifery education has improved. Although more and more graduate midwives are entering the profession, many find that they are unable to have some control over their work, use their skills, and make decisions. They encounter a working environment that is hostile and blame-seeking. Midwives are set against midwives, and intimidation and 'horizontal violence' is prevalent.[17–19] It is very difficult for midwives to continue to give supportive care to women when they themselves feel unsupported.

But this is not all. Mavis Kirkham, Professor of Midwifery at Sheffield University, tells me: 'The problem with midwifery is bureaucracy. Midwives get totally disillusioned and leave as practice gets rule-driven. We are all policing each other. It is not medical oppression. It is *bureaucratic* oppression. Midwives are supposed to be autonomous. But we are caught in a bureaucratic trap'. The depressing

Table 15.1 Examples of midwifery interventions in the second stage of labour

No intervention	First-level interventions	Second-level interventions	Third-level interventions
Woman remains in/moves to whatever position she chooses (with an open choice of positions available to her)	Asking a woman to change position, typically into an upright position	Asking a woman to push actively with contractions (but without breath-holding)	Swabbing or cleansing the vulval area
Woman bears down as and when she wants	Positively reinforcing woman's spontaneous pushing behaviour with encouraging words	Placing warm compresses on the perineum	Performing a vaginal examination to confirm full dilatation or to ascertain descent
Midwife guards and 'holds' a safe area around her until the baby is born	–	Cleaning away faeces from the perineal area	Catheterisation
–	–	Asking a woman to maintain a position where the midwife can see the woman's vulva	Performing manual vaginal distension to enlarge the birth canal

– Maintaining light counterpressure on the fetal head to slow down a rapid birth	Encouraging a woman to inhale, hold her breath and bear down strongly
– Asking a woman to 'pant' or 'blow' to slow down a rapid birth	Putting a woman into lithotomy or similar position
– Asking a woman if there are any psychological reasons why she is 'holding back'	'Guarding' the perineum and performing the Ritgen manoeuvre to deliver the head by controlled flexion and extension
– Massage of woman's legs and thighs to relax perineal area	Performing an episiotomy to expedite the birth

Table 15.2 Examples of midwifery interventions in the third stage of labour

No intervention	First-level interventions	Second-level interventions	Third-level interventions
Woman remains in/moves to whatever position she chooses	Asking a woman to change position, typically adopting an upright posture	Feeling the fundus to assess whether the placenta is separated; visualising signs of separation, such as cord lengthening	Asking the woman or her partner to stimulate her nipples to release oxytocin
Woman does whatever she chooses with the baby; picks it up as and when she wishes	Encouraging the woman to have 'skin-to-skin' contact with the baby	Asking a woman to push actively with contractions; woman delivers placenta	Active management of the third stage: giving an artificial oxytocin (e.g. syntrometrine); using controlled cord traction; midwife delivers placenta
Midwife guards and 'holds' a safe area around woman until placenta is out	Suggesting a woman puts the baby to lick/suckle at the breast	Asking the woman to cough, blow into a bag, etc.	Using complementary therapies, e.g. shiatsu points, homeopathic remedies, herbs

–	Drying, warming and/or wrapping the baby	Asking a woman to 'let go' of her placenta; asking her whether there is any psychological reason why she is 'holding on' to her placenta	Catheterisation
–	Ensuring the room is warm	Suggesting the woman sits on the toilet: to try to pass urine and sit upright in a familiar position	–
–	–	Pulling gently on the cord to deliver a separated placenta	–

conclusion may be drawn that, rather than eastern European midwifery being transformed to the standard of midwifery accepted in western European countries, in Britain midwifery is at risk of being degraded to conform with the totalitarian eastern European model.

References

1. Foster J, Anderson A, Houston, et al 2004 A report of a midwifery model for training traditional midwives in Guatemala. Midwifery: An International Journal 20(3):220

2. Stromerova Z 2002 Royal College of Midwives International Conference, Vienna. October

3. World Health Organisation 2003 Profiling midwifery in newly independent states and countries of central and eastern Europe. Geneva: WHO

4. Papp Z 2002 Statement of the Board of Hungarian Obstetricians and Gynaecologists on home birth. Budapest, Hungary, January

5. Statement of the Board of Hungarian Obstetricians and Gynaecologists on home birth. Budapest, Hungary, February 1999

6. Thomas M 2003 The crest of the wave – will midwives ride it? MIDIRS Midwifery Digest 13:3

7. Page L, Beake S, Viaol A 2001 Clinical outcomes of one-to-one midwifery practice. British Journal of Midwifery 9(11):700–706

8. Boulton M, Chapple J, Saunder D 2003 Evaluating a new service: clinical outcomes in women's assessment of the Edgware Birth Centre. In: Kirkham M (ed) Birth centres: a social model for maternity care. Oxford: Elsevier Science

9. Edwards NP 2001 Women's experiences of birthing autonomy: planning home births in Scotland. Unpublished PhD thesis, University of Sheffield

10. Haggerty JL, Reid RJ, Freeman GK, et al 2003 Continuity of care: a multidisciplinary review. BMJ 327(7425):1219–1221

11. Waldenstrom U, Turnbull D 1998 A systematic review comparing continuity of midwifery care with standard maternity services. British Journal of Obstetrics and Gynaecology 105(11):1160–1170

12. Page LA 2000 The new midwifery: science and sensitivity in practice. London: Elsevier Harcourt, p 123

13. Page LA 2000 The new midwifery: science and sensitivity in practice. London: Elsevier Harcourt, p 136

14. Department of Health 2003 NHS maternity statistics, England: 2001/2002. Bulletin 2003/09. London: DoH

15. Ashcroft B, Elstein M, Boreham N, et al 2003 Prospective semi-structured observational study to identify risk attributable to staff deployment, training, and updating opportunities for midwives. BMJ 327(7415):584

16. Anderson T 2002 Peeling back the layers: a new look at midwifery interventions. MIDIRS Midwifery Digest 12(2):207–210

17. Fanon F 1963 The wretched of the Earth. New York: Grove Press

18. Leap N 1997 Making sense of 'horizontal violence' in midwifery. British Journal of Midwifery 5:689

19. Ball L, Curtis P, Kirkham M 2002 Why do midwives leave? London: Royal College of Midwives

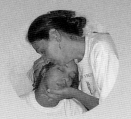

16
Doulas

An inexorable effect of the reduction in one-to-one midwife care over the last 35 years, intensified by integration of the midwifery services that has sucked midwives into hospital, means that few women get to know 'their' midwife and can think of her as a confiding friend. The diminution of community midwifery, combined with major social changes – smaller families and increased geographic mobility – has left many women isolated, without loving human support as they go through pregnancy, birth and new motherhood. The virtual loss of community midwifery over much of the UK has resulted in care being fragmented. In spite of there being a 'named' midwife on the case records, in practice a woman encounters members of a large team of midwives. She may find it difficult to put names to faces, and recoils from recounting her most personal details and private feelings and from being physically exposed to a virtual stranger. In childbirth it is stressful to have to handle fleeting relationships with professional caregivers who come and go and do not know you as an individual, are unaware of your hopes, fears and wishes, and for whom you are an allotted work task, rather than a person with your own identity.

However hard they try, a procession of different members of staff cannot give the warm glow of supportive human contact. It is impossible for the mother to be 'grounded'. She is confused and set adrift, a rudderless boat tossing in a stormy sea. Anne Enright, in her book *Making Babies*,[1] describes the effect of this during labour:

> *The door opens like an ordinary door. People come through it. First the student midwife, full of chat, then the midwife, fast and effective (it is in a hurry, this baby); she organises the epidural and then works on me, doing – I don't know*

what; it feels as if someone is taking a light bulb out of a too-narrow shade. After her, the Sister in charge, easy and reassuring. Then the consultant, who stares a little fixedly at the business end. Waking up. It is 3.00 a.m. Who will come in next? The master of the hospital, the Minister for Health, and then perhaps, God, as the baby puts its head out to taste the air.[1]

In the USA research shows that in some hospitals labour nurses only spend 6% of their time on duty giving support to women in childbirth. The rest of the time they are writing up notes, tending equipment, doing investigations, interacting with colleagues, clearing up and busying themselves with other chores. There simply is no time to be 'with woman'.[2] This is a problem throughout North America, and perhaps it is one of the reasons the caesarean rate in the USA rose to 27.6% in 2003.[3] In the UK midwifery is threatened by the same institutionalisation, bureaucratisation and fragmentation.

Many midwives make valiant efforts to provide sensitive, continuing care, but, as we have seen, it is often impossible because of the conditions under which they work and a system of management that turns them into cogs in a machine which, at all costs, must be kept running smoothly.

There is striking evidence that support from another woman during and after birth enhances the experience for the mother, makes birth safer for both her and her baby, and the transition to parenthood much more satisfying. This is why doulas have arrived on the scene. They give the intimate personal care that midwives now find it so hard to offer. The term 'doula' was first introduced by Dana Raphael, a social anthropologist who wrote a book about breastfeeding, and borrowed the term from the ancient Greeks, for whom it meant 'female slave' or 'handmaiden'.[4]

A doula is a trained and paid companion to a woman during birth and may attend her in her home through the first days or weeks after. She may be only a birth doula or only a postpartum doula, or may offer both these services. The essence of what doulas have to offer is summed up as 'social support'. It is not medical, although it overlaps with the art of midwifery. A doula draws on her knowledge of birth, and different kinds of birth, and of breastfeeding to give information so that women can come to their own decisions, provides emotional support and physical help, and enables everyone involved to communicate smoothly. She supports the partner and other members of the family, too, makes tea and coffee, clears up as she goes along, empties waste bins, cooks a delicious meal and cooperates with other helpers, including the partner, so that the woman is the focus of loving attention and can concentrate on the energy pouring through her body during labour. She may have other skills, including massage, aromatherapy, acupuncture or acupressure, reflexology or homeopathy, but the essence of what she offers is friendship and quiet confidence. She multi-tasks, remembering all the time that she is there for the woman and follows her guidance.[5]

Fourteen controlled trials around the world have produced remarkably consistent results regarding such support, in spite of different kinds of obstetric practice and birth environments, whether women were classified as high or low risk, and in situations where there were a mixed variety of professional caregivers and different policies about the presence of 'significant others'.[6]

There is strong research evidence to show that continuous support in childbirth reduces the use of pain-relieving drugs and lowers the epidural rate. It makes stimulation of labour with artificial oxytocin less likely, shortens labour, reduces the likelihood of forceps or vacuum extraction, cuts the caesarean section rate,[7] reduces the chance that the baby may have health problems after birth and need to go to the special care nursery,[8] reduces fever and infection in the mother and bleeding after childbirth, and reduces levels of anxiety and postpartum depression. Mothers have a more positive experience of birth and feel more in control.[9] Having a doula increases the chances of breastfeeding successfully, even when there has been no discussion about breastfeeding.[10] In fact, there is also some evidence that mothers show increased sensitivity towards their newborn babies.

More than any other intervention made in childbirth in the last 50 years, the introduction of a person who gives uninterrupted support and helps the woman be *heureuse dans sa peau* (happy in her own skin) has been shown to cut the rate of operative deliveries and to help make birth normal.

It is cost-saving too. In one hospital where a randomised control trial of doula care was carried out, the caesarean section rate was reduced by 10% and epidurals by 75% when women had doulas.[11, 12] It has been worked out that this alone is a massive cost-saving exercise and that if all women had doulas throughout childbirth the annual maternity healthcare costs in the USA would be reduced by more than $2 billion.[13, 14]

In an overview of the effects of doula support, a Professor of Obstetrics, a Professor of Midwifery and a doula who heads a doula training and consulting agency, state: 'Balancing the use of technology and medicine with the traditional ways of support returns nurturing, respect, and support to childbearing women and their partners. In today's birth experience, "high touch" complements "high tech"'.[15] They are very careful to avoid criticising high-tech obstetrics and seek to draw support from hospital obstetricians and management. In effect, they are saying that hiring doulas makes good business sense.

The conclusion of the Cochrane Systematic Review of randomised trials is: 'Given the clear benefits and no known risk associated with intrapartum support, every effort should be made to ensure that all labouring women receive support, not only from those close to them, but also from specially trained caregivers. This support should include continuous presence, the provision of hands-on comfort and encouragement'.[16]

In the USA, doulas are increasingly employed by hospitals. This may seem a cheap alternative to employing midwives and is less likely to threaten the status of obstetric nurses. It could have the effect of retarding the already slow regeneration of midwifery in North America. But, because doulas focus on serving women, it could also signal the need for midwives. If a doula can help make birth safer and more satisfying, how much more could midwives bring to childbirth in the USA?

But it is not that simple. When continuous support is provided by obstetric nurses – not doulas – who are already inculcated in routine practices in a high-tech hospital, one-to-one care may be far less effective than hoped. A randomised control trial was conducted in 13 North American hospitals in which 62% of labours were induced or augmented with oxytocin, 77% of women had continuous monitoring and 75% had regional anaesthesia.[17] The nurses were given a 2-day training in offering one-to-one support. The results were depressing. The power of the institutional environment proved overwhelming. It did not reduce the caesarean section rate and had no effect on any other medical or psychosocial outcome.

Doulas and midwives in the UK

The Royal College of Midwives (RCM) states that it 'supports women's choices in engaging the services of a doula due to an absence of social support traditionally provided by the family and believes that doulas may have a place as the woman's companion in labour or as a supporter/helper in the postnatal period'.[18] But the RCM 'opposes the employment of doulas in the maternity services', and prefers to engage maternity care assistants to work under the supervision of midwives. It warns: 'Doulas should not be used as substitutes for midwives'. This reflects a vigorous debate that is taking place among midwives. Doulas are on trial.

In the UK, doulas are skating on thin ice in their relations with midwives.[19] It is only too easy to confront, or take over – or simply make a midwife feel undervalued. It is equally easy for a midwife to come over to a doula as bossy or unfriendly. It is vital that each of them focus on the fact that they are there to serve the woman and her needs. A midwife who is herself also working as a doula comments that: 'Where the midwifery profession has to a large extent been complacent in its surrender to obstetric nursing, perhaps the rise of the doula is the very issue that will expedite the creation of a formal distinction between midwife and obstetric nurse?'[20]

Mary Cronk is an experienced midwife working mainly in the community. She has major reservations about the concept and the principle behind the doula movement. Years ago, working in Scotland, she said that there were always female companions, such as mums, aunties, cousins, friends and neighbours. 'They were invaluable. They fetched and carried, made me tea, supported my clients, made a contribution to good outcomes. They didn't think of themselves as doing anything special. They also supported me as a midwife'. Doulas are very different. 'They talk about "my client"' and, she believes, 'are saying to women that they know better than the midwife'. She describes how her advice to a woman who was in very early labour would be 'Keep your batteries charged. Get some sleep'. But a doula who had been to Active Birth classes told the mother, 'Keep active' and got her running up and down stairs. Mary went on to say, 'Those in charge of health service budgets welcome the doula with open arms because you can have a doula at half the price. Even better, she can be paid by the woman. Doulas are a threat to my profession. They stand in the way of what we want, which is more well-educated midwives'.

Debby Gould, Head of Midwifery and Gynaecology at St George's Hospital, London, also believes that doulas 'are a threat to the care that women receive'. Her greatest fear is that doulas will be incorporated within the National Health Service (NHS) system and employed by hospitals. Then the doula could no longer be truly a woman's advocate. 'Eventually they would start working 8-hour shifts and be equivalent to less well trained healthcare support workers. Doulas must be outside the system so they cannot be disciplined by it'. Doula UK, the main organisation of doulas in Britain, thinks the same. The doula should be the employee of the woman.

Debby described to me how midwives can feel sidelined by doulas. A midwife arrived on the scene when a woman was in labour, attended by her doula, and started asking her questions to find out when labour had started, how strong contractions were, whether her membranes had ruptured, and so on. The doula said: 'Talk to me – not to her. She needs to concentrate on her labour'. Debby says: 'I can see where the doula was coming from. You don't want to disturb the woman. But the midwife needed this information. Then the doula asked the midwife to go out of the room, which she did. The baby's head was born while she was outside. The woman wanted a physiological third stage and the doula covered her with a blanket and asked the midwife to leave her alone. The midwife, however, wanted to watch for blood loss. Not being able to see it, and not having been present at the birth of the baby made her subject to risk management'. The midwife had to explain to her managers why she did not carry out the duties of a midwife.

Conflicts like this can only be solved when midwives and doulas get together to discuss their roles and responsibilities. Doula UK is well aware of this and organises discussion groups and forums for midwives and doulas so that they can understand each other and work together better.

There are midwives who deflect their anxiety about being displaced by bureaucrats, technicians, managers and committees into hostility toward the easiest person to attack, someone lower in the pecking order. It could be a student midwife, a junior midwife, a doula, or even the patient herself. They can feel belittled and humiliated when a woman's primary relationship is with her doula instead of them. Rather than rejoicing that the woman is in a warm and supportive relationship, which has the potential to enhance her ability to trust her body and give birth spontaneously, these midwives feel threatened. They have often been swallowed up by a system that is impossible for them to control, however bravely they struggle. They may work hard to gain a woman's trust and to develop a unique relationship, only then to find that they are not wanted.

The Doula UK Code of Practice states that a doula offers support, but not advice, exploring options, and enabling the woman to make her own decisions: 'wherever and however she chooses to give birth. This may be home/birth centre/hospital, with or without medical interventions, whilst a postnatal doula supports the mother whether breast or bottle-feeding'.

'A doula does not perform clinical or medical tasks, diagnose medical conditions or give medical advice, even if trained as a health professional prior to becoming/ whilst practising'. If she is 'qualified as a therapist in some other field and wishes to apply this skill to her practice, it must be made clear that they are separate roles'. She 'will refer clients to other appropriate resources/professionals should the client have needs beyond the scope of the doula role'.

Doulas 'show integrity and respect at all times towards their clients, doula colleagues and other professionals with whom they may be working' and 'will not discuss personal and confidential information which has been disclosed to them by their clients' without their permission'.

In the USA the Standards of Practice of DONA (Doulas of North America) is explicit about interaction between doulas and professionals in the health services: 'The doula advocates for the client's wishes as expressed in her birth plan, in prenatal conversations, and intrapartum discussions, by encouraging her client to ask questions of her caregiver and express her preferences and concerns'. A doula 'enhances the communication between the client and caregivers. Clients and doulas must recognise that the advocacy role does not include the doula speaking instead of the client or making decisions for the client. The advocacy role is best described as support, information, and mediation or negotiation'. It seems to me that this extra clause could be an important addition to the UK Code of Practice.

But 'doulaing' should not be called a profession in the UK. Although some doulas are very experienced, it implies vigorous training over a period of years (not days).There is now, however, a regulatory body that sets standards, handles complaints, can strike off unsatisfactory members, and reward excellence.

The doula has a *vocation* to which she commits herself. She draws on her own life experience and knowledge of how women feel, and what help they need at times of crisis in their lives. She brings age-old skills and understanding from a community of women who always helped at and around birth. She needs to be quick to observe, respond, share, to know what she does not know, and to respect the experience of and autonomy of other women, including midwives.

What should a doula learn?

The core curriculum for any doula who is accredited by Doula UK includes obvious subjects, such as birth physiology, deviations from the norm, writing a birth plan, the needs of the mother and baby in the first 6 weeks, breastfeeding and bottle-feeding, and communication and listening skills. A doula empowers women to make informed choices and gives support rather than coaching. The curriculum also centres on the relationship between doulas and midwives, on knowledge of local protocols and the policy of service providers, and on being aware of other sources of support for the doula and sources of support for the family once the doula has left. Doulas learn how to intervene in a positive way when labour is not straightforward, by suggesting different postures, movements and breathing and giving the mother comfort. The focus is on 'creating a safe space rather than giving medical advice'. In the postpartum period a doula gives 'practical help which empowers the woman to do it for herself rather than having it done for her. The doula should make herself dispensable rather than indispensable'.

In the USA learning to be a doula entails attending a childbirth education course approved by the DONA Education Committee, reading four books from the DONA reading list and submitting an essay on the value and purpose of birth support. A doula must also support at least three clients, submit evaluations from clients and healthcare providers, together with records and descriptions of three births, and following certification she must be reassessed after each 3-year period of practice.

In the UK, doula organisations have mushroomed and each has its own approach. But to become recognised by Doula UK, a woman needs to sign a statement about the philosophy and Code of Practice, submit four client response forms concerning births she has attended or postnatal work she has done, and then be interviewed on a one-to-one basis by an assessor, who is herself an experienced doula.

A birth doula friend

Most research into the effects of having a birth companion have examined situations in which the companion is unknown to the mother before she goes into labour. We can guess that having someone with you who is already a friend may be even more effective. In the UK doulas get to know women in pregnancy, discuss their plans and wishes, find out exactly what they hope for from doula companionship, and meet the woman's partner, any other children, and often other members of the family too.

We did not call them doulas, but in the early days of National Childbirth Trust (NCT) teacher training the students I was tutoring not only attended a course of the classes I ran, but also accompanied at least one woman who was in that class when she was in labour, and I made arrangements with the largest hospital in the area so that this could become an accepted routine. It struck me then that this was an essential element in learning to be an antenatal teacher.

Being with a woman and her partner as she goes through childbirth classes, with all the discussions that take place about emotions and relationships, is equally important for a doula if she is to give of her best. It is not just that the novice doula is acquiring knowledge from the antenatal classes, exploring different positions and movements and rhythms of breathing for labour and birth, for example, she is sharing a journey with the woman through the pregnancy.

Where it is possible for a doula to get to know the midwife who is likely to attend the mother she is going to support, this is valuable too. They need to 'get on the same wavelength' and to understand what they expect from each other. I have had some doulas phone me in distress after a birth in which they were at loggerheads with a midwife, and we have tried to analyse together what went wrong and why. Nearly always conflict could have been avoided if the two had met and talked together earlier, meeting as colleagues who could help each other, and respecting the other's role, rather than being potential adversaries. However aggrieved a midwife or a doula may have been when there was hostility, they should remember that it is the birthing woman who suffered from it most. Where a midwife and doula work harmoniously together, they give something of inestimable value to a woman – they create an environment infused with peace, love and joy.

Maternity care assistants

Maternity care assistants are distinct from doulas. In The Netherlands they assist the midwife at the 30% of births that take place at home and, whether or not a woman gives birth at home, an assistant cares for mother and baby for 8 days and looks after the house and other children. In 73% of all births a maternity assistant is funded partly by government health insurance. Maternity care assistants have 4 months' training and work under supervision for a year.

A randomised controlled trial of maternity care assistants for 28 days after birth in the UK, based on the Dutch model, revealed that, although women liked it, there were no differences in rates of depression, physical health, breastfeeding or the use of the NHS.[21] Maybe all this official support disempowered women from finding their own support network.[22] On the other hand, some birth centres are using maternity care assistants very successfully. The assistants are responsible to the midwife, care for the woman and her baby, assist in emergencies, and do clerical work, housekeeping and help with antenatal classes and postnatal groups.[23]

Some of these assistants, like some doulas, go on to train as midwives. It should be recognised as a career pathway, especially for women who, perhaps because their educational qualifications do not enable them to enter midwifery training directly, have the right personality to do this work. Professor Jane Sandall of King's College Hospital points out that 'the training of healthcare assistants working in maternity care is of variable quality across the country. Currently, it is too focused on the needs of the hospital rather than women; it is not designed for working in the community or specifically for maternity care. It is also essential that it provides pathways into midwifery education and that it positively encourages women from ethnic minorities and socially disadvantaged groups to work in this field. European social fund money which provides equal opportunities for such women could be used for this'.[23] She goes on to say that it would be wrong to welcome assistants simply to 'plug gaps in an alienating dehumanising system'. Offering genuine friendship, engendering self-confidence, and giving time, are some of the most precious attributes for anyone in the maternity services who aims to provide woman-centred care.

Mothers on postnatal wards often feel totally neglected. Time and time again I hear from women who have had initial problems breastfeeding say, 'Thank heavens for the cleaner! She had breastfed her own children and showed me how to do it'; 'The cleaner told me that everyone where she came from breastfed and she gave me confidence'; or 'The nurses were so busy that they didn't have time to help me get him sucking happily, but there was a cleaner who showed me how to hold him so that he could latch on easily and how to know when the sucking and swallowing showed he was feeding well'.

At present, with midwives absorbed by the medical system, trying to do many technical tasks that used to be done by doctors, and spending much of their time filling in forms, it is often ancillary staff who give emotional support and practical help to women on postnatal wards. Nurturing women through the all-important first days of the transition to motherhood and providing care that is humane and empowering during childbirth should not be left to chance. Women, together with the midwives who care for them, need uninterrupted support and validation of their value and identity.

References

1. Enright A 2004 Making babies: stumbling into motherhood. London: Jonathan Cape, Random House, p 91

2. Gagnon AJ, Waghorn K 1996 Supportive care by maternity nurses: a work sampling study in an intrapartum unit. Birth 23(1):1–6

3. Hamilton BE, Martin JA, Sutton PD 2004 Births: preliminary data for 2003. National vital statistics reports, vol 53, No. 9. Hyattsville, MD: National Center for Health Statistics. Available at: http://www.cdc.gov/nchs (accessed November 2004)

4. Raphael D 1976 The tender gift: breastfeeding. New York: Schocken Books

5. Hodnett ED 2000 Caregiver support for women during childbirth. Cochrane Database Systematic Review 2:CD000199. Update: Cochrane Database Systematic Review 2002;1:CD000199

6. Enkin M, Keirse M, Neilson J, et al 2000 A guide to effective care in pregnancy and childbirth, 3rd edn. Oxford: Oxford University Press

7. Scott KD, Berkowitz G, Klaus M 1999 A comparison of intermittent and continuous support during labor: a meta-analysis. American Journal of Obstetrics and Gynecology 180(5):1054–1059

8. Kennell J, Klaus M, McGrath S, et al 1991 Continuous emotional support during labor in a US hospital. A randomized trial. JAMA 265:2197–2201

9. Scott KD, Klaus PH, Klaus MH 1999 The obstetrical and postpartum benefits of continuous support during childbirth. Journal of Women's Health and Gender Based Medicine 8:1257–1264

10. Campero L, Garcia C, Diaz C, et al 1998 'Alone, I wouldn't have known what to do': a qualitative study on social support during labor and delivery in Mexico. Social Science and Medicine 47:395–403

11. Langer A, Campero L, Garcia C, Reynoso S 1998 Effects of psychosocial support during labour and childbirth on breastfeeding, medical interventions, and mothers' wellbeing in a Mexican public hospital: a randomised clinical trial. British Journal of Obstetrics and Gynaecology 105:1056–1063

12. Klaus MH, Kennell JH 1997 The doula: an essential ingredient of childbirth rediscovered. Acta Paediatrica 86:1034–1036

13. Kennell J, Klaus M, McGrath S, et al 1991 Continuous emotional support during labor in a US hospital. A randomized trial. JAMA 265:2197–2201

14. Klaus M, Kennell J, Berkowitz G, Klaus P 1992 Maternal assistance and support in labor: father, nurse, midwife or doula? Clinics in Consulting Obstetrics and Gynecology 4:211–217

15. Meyer BA, Arnold JA, Pascali-Bonaro D 2001 Social support by doulas during labor and the early postpartum period. Hospital Physician September:57–65

16. Hodnett ED 2000 Caregiver support for women during childbirth. Cochrane Database Systematic Review 2:CD000199 Update: Cochrane Database Systematic Review 1:CD000199

17. Hodnett ED, Lowe NK, Hannah ME, et al 2002 Effectiveness of nurses as providers of birth labor support in North American hospitals: a randomised control trial. JAMA 288(11):1373–1381

18. Royal College of Midwives 2004 Position statement 6. Doulas. London: RCM. Available at: http://www.rcm.org.uk/data/info_centre/data/position_papers.htm (accessed November 2004)

19. Mander R 2002 Is the doula merely an answer to an obstetrician's prayer? MIDIRS Midwifery Digest 12(1):8–12

20. Stockton A 2003 Doulas – the future guardians of normal birth? MIDIRS Midwifery Digest 13(3):347–350

21. Morrell CJ, Spibey H, Stuart P, et al 2001 Costs and benefits of community post natal support. MIDIRS Midwifery Digest 11(4):550

22. Sandall J 2001 Extending the establishment – maternity assistant or doulas? MIDIRS Midwifery Digest 11(4):547–550

23. Saunders D, Bolton M, Chappell J et al 2000 Evaluation of the Edgware Birth Centre. Harrow: Perinatal Public Health, Northwick Park Hospital, North Thames

17
Fathers

In many cultures childbirth, like menstruation, is thought to bring danger to men who encroach too near. In Judaeo-Christian thought, this idea can be traced back to Leviticus. The 7th-century Archbishop Theodore of Canterbury proclaimed that a newly delivered woman must be isolated for 40 days until clean, and that if any woman went into a church while menstruating she had to fast for 3 weeks. The Penitential of Archbishop Egber 766 AD states that 'every religious woman should keep her chastity for 3 months before childbirth and for 60 nights and days after'. This is not for the woman's sake, but because a newly delivered woman is dangerous to men. Not only is the menstruating and parturient woman ritually unclean, but her body products, nail parings, hair clippings and, most important of all, her secretions and blood, are taboo to men, and can result in their illness or death.

There is a strict rule in many cultures that the father should stay away from the place of birth. Male and female elements must be kept separate. But, even when he is not supposed to be there, it is often believed that the baby's health and life depend on the father's actions. He has a ritual responsibility to ensure a safe pregnancy and birth. If he goes off with another woman, or even polishes his spear, or goes fishing on the day of labour, he is putting the baby's life at risk. He must conduct himself with care, and in this way help the birth. So he participates actively, even though he is not physically present. The Koran states that a father should offer prayers at birth, and he introduces the baby to the world by placing a piece of date in its mouth.

The Arapesh of New Guinea rely on the prospective father to contribute towards the health and welfare of the unborn baby by his careful conduct, both in the way that he has intercourse – deliberately and thoughtfully in the early weeks of pregnancy – and in the emotionally supportive, stress-free environment he should create for the pregnant woman. In fact, in New Guinea the verb 'to bear a child' applies equally to women and men, and childbearing is believed to be as much a strain for the father as it may be for the mother. He is involved from the very beginning of pregnancy, because the Arapesh believe that a man must really work at sexual intercourse in order for a child to be conceived, and continue doing this until his wife's periods stop. But once her breasts begin to enlarge the child is complete in miniature, and from then on intercourse is forbidden.

In Thailand it is the father's responsibility to cut and stack the tamarind wood ready for the mother's 'fire-rest' after childbirth when she lies on a board near a fire that protects her from evil spirits. In northern Thailand he must also build a fence around the area under the house, which is built on stilts, directly under the birth room, and place thorns all around this fence to keep out evil spirits. After the baby is born he cooks for his wife for the first 2 weeks or so.

In the few societies where the husband catches the baby himself, as he does among the Bang Chan of south-east Asia, he must be specially protected from female forces. He takes incense, flowers and a lighted candle, which allow him to cross over into the sacred world in which birth takes place. Then he prays for the help of the spirits to make the winds of birth strong in his body, for it is not he but the winds which deliver the baby, and he is there only to receive it.

The couvade

In the custom of the *couvade*, from the French 'to hatch', the husband either shares in the birth by acting it out at the same time as his wife is in labour, or he shares the lying-in period. Especially in societies in which it is uncertain who exactly the father of the baby is, this is a way in which a man claims fatherhood. An Arapesh father, for example, waits to hear the sex of the baby. Then he says 'wash it' or 'do not wash it', depending on whether he wishes it to live or not. In many societies, abortion or infanticide are the only effective means of birth control, and boys are usually preferred because they will grow up to inherit their father's land, while girls will pass outside the paternal family. It is the father who makes the decision.

The Arapesh father takes a bundle of soft leaves to his wife so that she can line the net bag in which the baby is suspended in a crouching position, a coconut shell of water for bathing the baby, and pungent leaves to keep evil out of her hut. He also brings his wooden pillow and lies down beside his wife. Both have nothing to eat or drink for the first day after birth. They concentrate on performing magic rites for the welfare of the child and remain in seclusion for 5 days. The father must not touch his own body or handle tobacco. He must eat all food with a spoon until a ceremony of ritual cleansing is performed at a pool in a leaf house built beside it. Even then, his diet is still restricted, and he cannot eat meat until the baby is a month old.

In Mediterranean cultures the father may be required by the midwife to assist by enacting rites to help the progress of labour. In peasant Greece, for example, if labour is long she asks him to unknot his tie and undo all buttons so that labour may be freed. Water may also be poured through his shirt sleeves to symbolise the flow of birth. In Jamaica, the *nana* seeks to stimulate a uterus that is not contracting well by getting the mother to take deep breaths of the sweat on his shirt, a rite that may have the effect of stimulating labour through the action of prostaglandins.

Fathers in Europe and North America

Historically, in western Europe fathers rarely attended birth, except in The Netherlands.

Writing about birth in the East End of London in the 1950s, a midwife says:

> *When everything was shipshape, the proud father was permitted to enter. These days, most fathers are with their wives throughout labour, and attend the birth ... In the 1950s everyone would have been profoundly shocked at such an idea. Childbirth was considered to be a woman's business ... I regretted ... that I could not get to know the men of the East End. But it was quite impossible. I belonged to the women's world, the taboo subject of childbirth. The men were polite and respectful to us midwives, but completely withdrawn from any familiarity, let alone friendship. There was a total divide between what was called men's work and women's work. So, like Jane Austin, who in all her writing never recorded a conversation between two men alone, because she as a woman could not know what exclusively male conversation could be like, I cannot record much about the men of Poplar ...*[1]

In northern industrial countries fathers started to be involved in childbirth in the 1970s, largely because, with the switch from home to hospital, female support groups had disappeared. Women helpers were not allowed to be present in hospital, and even if a woman in labour pleaded for her mother or sister to attend, it might not be permitted. Hospital midwives were anxious that they would lose control if the patient's relatives and friends were allowed in.

In the UK it was rare for fathers to be present until the first middle-class fathers were invited into the delivery room by obstetricians in the 1960s in a few of the large London teaching hospitals. The idea was that the father could give emotional support by sitting quietly beside the woman, although in at least one hospital this had to be in the corner of the room, so that he did not 'get in the way'.

I had already started the National Childbirth Trust (NCT) couples' birth classes held after working hours in the UK. NCT classes were usually held in the daytime and fathers were invited to attend only a special 'parents' evening'. Instead of this arrangement, I invited a woman to bring with her anyone whom she thought would be a good support person. It might be her male partner, another woman, her mother, or another relative. I also had a private consultation with each couple to explore emotional aspects of birth, parenthood and family relationships, sex, and other issues personal to them. In a modified form this gradually became part of NCT teaching generally, although hospital birth classes stuck with the 'parents' evening' style of antenatal teaching. Over time, NCT study days for National Health Service (NHS) midwives and physiotherapists succeeded in changing much of the teaching in hospitals too, and introduced the topic of the psychological experience for both parents.

In the USA, father involvement was still taboo at the start of the 1970s. Direct confrontation occurred in a Chicago hospital when a man chained himself to the delivery table, and could not be removed before the birth. Grudging acceptance of some fathers only came in the mid-1970s, after publication of *Thank you Dr Lamaze*, which promoted the system of psychoprophylaxis taught by Fernand Lamaze at the Clinique des Metallurgistes in Paris.[2] In France a woman was directed by her personal *monitrice*, a female obstetric physiotherapist. In the USA, the husband took her place. Some obstetricians welcomed the new liaison with fathers, and felt happier with another man in the room to help control the mother. Father participation came about only as an 'alternative' method. It entailed a direct challenge to the medical system. 'Husband coached' and drug-free childbirth was promoted by a maverick obstetrician, Robert Bradley.[3] He said that he was 'just a farm boy at heart' and had learned obstetrics by observing parturition in pigs.

The Bradley method put the husband firmly in charge of his wife. His task was to keep the woman under control. Bradley held 'rooster parties' for men, in which they were taught how to keep their wives quiet, contented and obedient during labour. The idea spread, and the male 'coach' replaced the female birth companion. This was one effect of the shrinking of the extended family to a much smaller group consisting only of a man and wife and their children, and it reinforced the man's conventional position of power vis-á-vis his wife.

When men become trainers birth is diminished by 'characterising it as a sport, a competition, over which men exercise a kind of playful authority (often supplemented by "funny" coach T-shirts or even commercial kits complete with coaching cap, digital stopwatch (to time contractions), sports bottle, counter-pressure ball, hyperventilation bag, time-of-delivery pool card, ear plugs and coaching tips for every phase of labor)'.[4]

The 'husband-coached' model of father participation is not so much evidence of the arrival of the 'new man', and of gender transformation, as a sign of the reinforcing of a traditional gender role.

The Bradley method has changed over the years. The emphasis now is on natural birth without drugs, rather than the dominant role of the male partner.

Michel Odent criticises father's involvement in birth for different reasons.[5] He believes that the man prevents the woman finding her 'primitive self', by intellectualising birth and even reducing it to a system of exercises. So he devises tasks for the father, such as electrical repairs or jobs in the kitchen, which remove him from the birth room. He writes: 'At the very time when the labouring woman needs to reduce the activity of her intellect (of her neocortex) and "to go to another planet", many men cannot stop being rational. Some look brave, but their release of high levels of adrenaline is contagious'.[6] He is critical also of the presence of friends and family. He thinks that, ideally, a woman should labour in the dark alone. If anyone is present, she should not be aware of it.

It is certainly the case that any system in which another person, whether lay or professional, manages labour and delivery and directs the women's behaviour risks turning childbirth into a performance, a display of skill, a competitive sport, or a test of womanhood. When a midwife takes on this managerial role she, too, is likely to intrude on the spontaneous and instinctive interaction of mind and body in childbirth.

Is there a role for the father in childbirth?

A couple can be drawn closer together by sharing the birth experience and the man can gain deeper understanding of his partner's needs, an understanding that stays with him so that he becomes more perceptive and empathetic generally, and in tune with the baby.

For this to happen, though, he must not take on the role of coach or teacher, but be there to do what his partner wants, and serve, if necessary, as interpreter or mediator between her and her professional attendants. This demands great sensitivity. On the other hand, sensitivity is not enough. The woman should not be made anxious about his emotional reactions. She has to be confident that he is strong enough to face the power of birth and the nakedness of human emotions as the birth energy sweeps through her body.

There are women who say, 'I couldn't have done it without him', and women who go out of labour when the man leaves to have a quick meal, just as there are women who can only labour well when the man is absent.

This is why it is important for a woman to think through the quality of support she needs and work it out with her partner well ahead of time. Her needs are paramount and his emotional reaction to being wanted or not wanted is of secondary importance.

Through her understanding, a midwife can facilitate discussion of these matters and enable the couple to communicate openly and honestly with each other.

References

1. Worth J 2002 Call the midwife. Twickenham: Merton Books, pp 14–15
2. Karmel M 1982 Thank you, Dr Lamaze, revised edn. London: HarperCollins
3. Bradley RA 1974 Husband-coached childbirth, revised edn. New York: Harper & Row, p 12

4. Pollock D 1999 Telling bodies, performing birth. Columbia, NY: Columbia University Press

5. Odent M 2002 The farmer and the obstetrician. London: Free Association Books

6. Odent M 2002 The farmer and the obstetrician. London: Free Association Books, p 98

18

Children at birth

When Josh, my grandson, was 5 years old, he came home from school with a worksheet about what babies can do at different ages. At birth they can suck. And there was a drawing of a newborn sucking – on a bottle. This was advance advertising of artificial baby milk to parents of the future.

Baby Hospital, a TV documentary screened in the early evening when children are likely to be glued to the screen, filmed a birth. The mother had an epidural, and since she was covered by drapes it was impossible to tell from where the baby was emerging. It could have been her umbilicus, or possibly her big toe. The midwife who took over from another when the shift changed, praised her for being an 'ideal patient – she was so calm'. Calm was not in it. Mildly disgruntled and irritated by what she was expected to do, she might have been putting on a tight shoe or pulling weeds. The baby was born, wrapped, and plonked on her chest. She gave it a cursory glance, but did not touch it, and continued to talk and look around the room. Because she was reclining, it would have been difficult for her to gaze into the baby's eyes. It was the father who, when handed the baby, looked down at her face and greeted her; and then the older sibling who walked in at that point.

This was birth without striving, without passion, without joy. It was an insidious way of teaching children that it entails some obscure kind of tricky work in the lower part of a woman's body, that it does not hurt, and other people do it for her.

A BBC film that is often used in schools is completely unsuitable for primary age children.[1] The language is medicalised, and the games that involve racing of sperm to ovum are geared to adolescent boys. Birth is summed up as uterine activity that 'painfully forces the cervix open'.

So when I consulted the Department of Education I was not surprised that a spokesperson told me that children aged 5–10 years are not learning much about emotions or relationships. They are taught biology. This tends to be delayed until the last year of primary school, since teachers rarely feel comfortable with it. There is a plethora of illustrations of cross-sections of body organs – the 'slice 'em up and explain what and where' approach to sex education.

In practice, children learn about birth almost exclusively from TV soaps and hospital situation comedies (sit-coms), in which birth is depicted as an emergency, with overtones of impending catastrophe, and final salvation by the obstetrician. They learn that birth means fear, a frantic rush to hospital, and life-saving surgery. I walked into the room to hear a distressed woman on a TV soap saying 'I'm having a baby! Call an ambulance!' We condition children to think of birth as like a road accident or a heart attack. This may be why many first-time mothers want to make sure that they can have an epidural as soon as they step through the hospital doors or opt for an elective caesarean.

It was not always like this. In the middle ages, Florentine and Sienese paintings of the birth of St. Mary and St. John sometimes showed children present, either playing, or helping the god-sibs, the female friends who attended the birth to care for the mother and baby. German woodcuts from the 16th century also show children at birth.[2]

But this had all changed by the 19th century. Victorians, or at least, members of the middle class, told children that the doctor brought the baby in his little black bag, or that it was plucked from under a gooseberry bush. Many girls grew up ignorant about where babies came from and how they got out. Death, in contrast, was considered highly suitable for children, and morally uplifting. They joined the mourning circle around the death bed, viewed the body, and made mourning cards. Isolating them from any knowledge about birth, however, and from the sexual implications of reproduction, was a sign of higher social status. While the poor lived in crowded hovels where birth was highly visible, those who had more money could shroud it in secrecy.

Yet in the 20th century, before most births in Britain took place in hospital following the Second World War, many children were around when a baby was born, although they might be sent off to Granny when delivery was

1 week

Part of a school worksheet given to my 5-year-old grandson

imminent, or she came to care for them in their own home. Some happened to be present at the birth and climbed on the bed to hold the new baby when only a few minutes old. They did not get any formal education, but birth was seen as a normal part of life. When birth was moved to the hospital, it was no longer an experience for the whole family, and it has generally remained that way.

Even when there is an opportunity to have children present, women sometimes tell me, 'I wouldn't want the children there. I'd hate them to see me in pain', and 'It's way beyond what a 3 year old can cope with emotionally. It might traumatise her for life'. Midwives may feel this way, too. Yet one midwife described with delight how when she was assisting at a birth, as the head was born the 3 year old jumped up on the bed, a gift-wrapped box in his hand, saying excitedly, 'Hello baby! Here's your birthday present!'

I wrote about this in a parenting column, and asked mothers to let me know children's reactions to being present at birth, and solicited drawings and tape-recorded or written accounts from their children. The result was 52 accounts from mothers and 35 drawings and accounts from young children. These were, with few exceptions, home births, and having the children there, if it worked out that way, was one of the reasons for women deciding to give birth at home. Children were also able to get to know the midwives in advance. As Catherine put it:

> From the moment when I (supported by partner and six wonderful midwives in a St. Thomas's group practice) chose a home birth I think Sophie assumed she would be there. She met all the midwives and came to most check-ups, taking it all in her stride, happily colouring in a picture whilst that amazing sound of the baby's heart beat suddenly filled the room. I realised we had to work into the plans for my labour fetching Sophie from school if she was inconveniently there. She insisted on it ... When we made our one single trip actually inside St. Thomas' for Sam's scan, Sophie came along.

It is important to prepare children so that they can understand what is happening. Not only about things that they will see, but also the sounds of birth:

> We looked at lots of pictures of newborn babies, of women in the late stages of labour, of umbilical cords and placentas in womb photos and diagrams. We watched Gaby's labour on Neighbours. It was very unreal, shot from the waist upwards literally, and yet had a degree of something I recognised – 'I can't do this now!' Afterwards Sophie asked why Gaby had been making 'funny noises'. Oops! I realised that although I had been concerned about pain I had forgotten this bit for Sophie and had concentrated on the delivery. So Sophie's preparation continued, with talks about strong muscles and hard work and pictures of women breathing and distracted.

One way of preparing children for the 'funny noises' is to act out breathing through contractions and the sounds of second-stage pushing. Small children often like to try this out, too, and it turns into a game. Catherine laboured during the night and when Sophie woke in the morning she 'heard noises', which she knew were signs of a baby on the way:

> David, my partner, had the presence of mind to mention in time that we wanted Sophie with us as I rested with my head in his lap, kneeling beside my bed. Rebecca (the midwife) immediately went to fetch her and she slipped into the room. She gave David a hug and sat on the floor between David and Rebecca. She remembers seeing Sam's head and I remember Rebecca saying "Your baby has dark hair Sophie" – a really reassuring remark. I was almost there! When Sam was born, first I held him, wrapped in a towel, umbilical cord still attached. David then held him and Sophie also, after asking to do so. David took photos and we also have one taken by Sophie (having a snappy camera of her own was one of our preparation points!).

> It was very natural that Sophie was there, in her parent's bedroom, to watch her brother coming into the world. It was very much her decision, but one that fit easily with, and probably partly came from, the type of birth we planned, and were supported in planning and hoping for by my midwife. Of course we discussed possible problems and alternative not-so-perfect scenarios. And having her with us was something that involved thought and careful preparation, but not unlike preparations I was making anyway in my own mind. I think if she hadn't been there I'd be now thinking 'If only ...!'

Sophie drew a picture of her mother holding newborn Sam in her lap, with her toy Dalmatian sitting beside them. She said:

> When I woke up I got out of my cot and got my 101 Dalmatians book and read it to my dog, Pongo. Then one of the midwives came in and said, "Your baby's being born". And then I went in and saw his head coming out. I stayed off school that day because I wanted to see Sam. I felt happy about him being born because I used to not have someone to play with, only Mummy and Daddy.

Typical accounts from mothers are:

> They came into the bedroom, cuddled me and asked me if they could watch a video in Tim's room while they waited. Off they went and they continued to pop back in and out. My husband fetched them as Daniel was about to emerge. The midwife asked Tim (7) if he wanted to hold the baby. He refused, saying he would wait till he had had a bath. As the midwife cleaned and checked Daniel over she asked the children to help by counting his fingers and toes. This made them feel important. The children sat next to me on the bed and Tim sang Happy Birthday to him. No-one had told him to do this. Jessica (5) held him and talked to him as if he could understand her ... The bond between them was instantaneous. They are both brilliant with Daniel.

Jason was 3 years old, and his mother wrote: 'He rubbed my back during contractions. After Molly was born he knelt down beside me and hugged me and said, "You got the baby out very well, Mummy"'. Harry was 2 years old, and:

'When Beth came out he was yelling "bubby, bubby!" He then helped cut the cord. Having him there helped me, as his presence kept me calm and more controlled. He was more than observer, as he helped by spraying me with water. He felt part of it. I wasn't sure how much of it he would remember, yet (8 months later) he still speaks about it. I feel that having him there helped him accept his sister. I haven't had the usual jealousy problems and he is very protective of Beth'.

Caroline wrote to me about her 4-year-old son, whom they 'included throughout the pregnancy so he knew our midwives and doctor and when I was in labour we explained that the baby was coming soon. (He rubbed my back during contractions and saw the whole birth.)'.

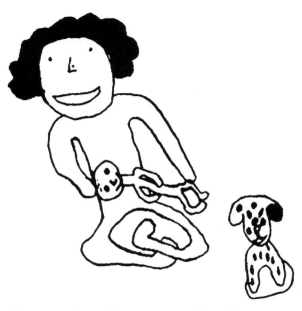

'Our new baby and Pongo my dog': Sophie's drawing

Three children said they did not like things about the birth, but were glad that they had been there. For the rest it was a very positive experience. Anna, now 13, wrote that when she was 6, 'I was lucky enough to see my younger sister Daisy being born. Her birth is one of my most vivid and exciting memories and I realise now that I was lucky being able to share that special day with my Mum, Dad and, of course, Daisy. During the 7 years that I have been her older sister we have shared a bond which has grown from me being at the birth. I am like a second mother to her. When Daisy wants Mummy she can turn to me as an alternative'. Eight-year-old Ashley wrote: 'Kate woke us up and took us to the hospital. It was very boring when Mummy was roaring and carrying on. After a little while I saw Hope's head. She had a lot of hair. When she came out she had a Martian head. [The baby was persistent posterior, with sugar-loaf moulding.] She was a bit goopey but I loved her anyway'.

Sarah, now 14, said about David's birth 18 months ago: 'I had to bring flannels because Mum was always too hot or too cold, to put them on her forehead and damp her wrists ... When he came out he was all covered in blood. I expected

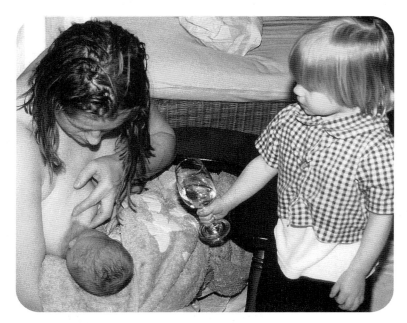

Birth is thirsty work. The older sister offers her mother a drink while she feeds the newborn

him to be clean like in the films. We were the first people he saw. It's a nice experience. I think children should be there'.

These children are fortunate. It is not only that they have acquired accurate information. They have shared in the excitement of labour, witnessed the spectacular power of women's bodies, and are aware of the impact that birth can have on emotions and relationships.

References

1. The human body, life stages. BBC Worldwide, 1988
2. Kitzinger S 2000 Rediscovering birth. London: Little Brown, pp 99–127

19

Silence is collusion: violence in pregnancy

Violence against women in pregnancy, misnomered 'domestic' violence, is given little social acknowledgement. It is, almost without exception, male violence. Caregivers often prefer not to see it, and have no idea what action to take if they do. To talk to women about it would be embarrassing and intrude on a couple's relationship, which is a matter for them alone. Although doctors, nurses and midwives tackle subjects such as sexually transmitted diseases, fetal abnormalities, miscarriage, preterm birth and perinatal mortality rates, this is the last taboo.

Internationally, statistics reveal that one in four women suffers 'domestic' violence at some time in her life.[1] Home Office figures in Britain show that every 3 days a woman is killed by her partner or ex-partner.[2] In pregnancy, violence is more common than conditions for which women are routinely screened, such as pregnancy-induced hypertension and diabetes.[3]

The Confidential Enquiry into Maternal Deaths[4] covering the period 1997–1999, revealed that 12% of the 378 women whose death was reported to the enquiry had told a healthcare professional about the violence to which they were subjected during their pregnancy. Since no women in the report had been specifically asked whether they were experiencing violence, 12% is most likely to be an underestimate. Of the girls under the age of 18 whose deaths came to the notice of the enquiry, 80% had suffered physical and/or sexual violence in their own home. All those who died aged 16 or under had been abused by a family member. Many women who spoke of violence booked late to attend the antenatal clinic, or did not attend. When interpreters were used, they were often male members of the family within which the abuse was experienced. Most women received little or no help to escape from violence.

A survey by Women's Aid revealed that only 27% of health authorities had written policies concerning domestic violence, although another 15% had agreed practice, but no written policy.[5] Only 9% of Primary Care Groups and Trusts had written policies.

Another study looked at policies and practice in maternity units.[6] Only 12% had a written policy, although another 30% had some kind of agreed practice. Less than 50% of the maternity units routinely offered a woman an antenatal appointment without her partner. There was a lack of printed information in places where women could read it in privacy, without the family member who was abusing them being aware of it. Just over 50% had printed information in the clinic, but only a quarter had information in the toilets. Only three units audited their domestic violence practices.[7] The Confidential Enquiry into Maternal Deaths stressed:

- the responsibility of all health professionals to be aware of the importance of domestic violence
- the development of local strategies and guidelines for the identification and support of women victims, including multi-agency working
- the provision of information in clinics about sources of help for victims
- that routine questions about violence be included in asking about social problems and that obstetricians and gynaecologists should ask all women about violence
- that all women are seen on their own at least once during their antenatal care
- that routine questioning must be accompanied by training for professionals and provisions for referral
- that, if needed, an interpreter should be provided, who should not be a partner, friend or family member.[7]

The National Perinatal Epidemiology Unit found that most women, both victims and non-victims, do not mind being asked about their experiences of violence, and expect caregivers to act on the information they give them. Drawing on women's own reports and suggestions, the recommendations they make for caregivers include:

- listening to women
- providing enough time and privacy
- asking directly about abuse
- responding with sympathy and understanding
- making clear that they reject domestic violence
- not blaming women or making a joke of the situation
- taking care about confidentiality and safety
- being well informed about abuse in general and local resources
- referring women appropriately
- not relying on medication as the response
- not being critical if a woman does not resolve the situation quickly.

One of the subjects that has not been researched is whether routine screening for violence could cause harm. It is very important to evaluate every project that is designed to uncover violence and protect women and children.

If enquiries by health professionals simply lead to increased referral to other agencies, little is achieved. In fact, the enquiry itself is potentially harmful because it may alert abusers and increase the violence. Studies of screening programmes are needed that assess their psychological effects, and their impact on the quality of life. It should not be assumed that screening leads to appropriate interventions and support. The National Perinatal Epidemiology Unit concluded that there was no evidence of the benefit of specific interventions, nor proof that screening could not be harmful.[8] These were the research questions they raised:

- What are the benefits and risks to women of screening for domestic violence in healthcare settings?
- What is the most effective screening interval?
- What is the effect of participation in interventions, such as provision of advocacy support, on women experiencing domestic violence identified in healthcare settings?
- What are the training needs of health professionals in relation to domestic violence?
- How can we promote better multi-agency working in this area?

It is not just a question of identifying women who are abused. What matters is the steps that are taken afterwards, and the effect on the women and their relationships.

Much of the violence against pregnant women and new mothers involves sexual abuse. In an interview the formerly feminist novelist Fay Weldon was asked why she stated that rape was not among the worst crimes. She replied, 'After all, it's only a penis'.[9] This ignores the context in which forced penetration occurs. I wonder what the woman whose partner tore out her episiotomy sutures in order to rape her would have thought about that. Trivialising rape means ignoring bite marks, the knife, the rope, the broken glass, hands that choke, and the tyranny of uncontrolled power. Violence may start postpartum, too, perhaps because a woman does not seem to belong to the man any longer, but to the baby. A Swedish study explored physical and sexual violence in the 8 weeks after childbirth. A random sample of women were asked whether they had experienced abuse. Of 132 women who answered the questionnaire, 32 reported threats, or physical or sexual abuse. Of these, 22 had not been subjected to this before the baby was born.[10]

The All-Parliamentary Group on Maternity, under the aegis of the National Childbirth Trust with the Royal College of Midwives, the Royal College of Obstetricians and various childbirth organisations, meets regularly in the House of Commons, and is attended by politicians of all parties. Working together, we succeeded in drawing attention to the alarming increase in the rate of caesarean sections and other obstetric interventions, and stimulated research into how to increase the proportion of normal births by ensuring that every woman is cared for by a midwife who knows how to support physiological birth. Meetings direct attention to political issues in birth that need to be dealt with at a parliamentary level. As a result, questions are asked in the House, investigative committees set up, legislative changes made, and public policy developed.

After Labour came to power in Britain, the National Health Service established a group to review murders in which domestic violence was a factor. It laid down policy and procedure guidelines. This followed the 1998 publication of the report *Why Mothers Die: Confidential Enquiries into Maternal Deaths*, which, for the first time, included deaths from violence.[11] A task group was set up and 4-day multi-agency training courses started, with caregivers in many different fields, and peer groups for ongoing support.

Representing the Lord Chancellor's department, the Solicitor General, Harriet Harman, spoke at a meeting of the Intra-Party Parliamentary Group, and told how one pregnant woman repeatedly went to her doctor with injuries. She was not asked anything about violence, and her relationship with her partner was never discussed. Subsequently, he murdered her and their two children.

The NHS has been the slowest of all agencies to tackle the subject of violence in pregnancy. Research shows that around 30% of abuse starts when a woman is pregnant, and that in an existing abusive relationship violence escalates with pregnancy,[12] although only 27% of health authorities have written policies about domestic violence, and less than half have a designated officer for tackling it.[13] The Royal College of Midwives and the Royal College of Obstetricians both now address the subject of male violence against women. But the Royal College of Psychiatrists has ignored the subject completely, although a large proportion of deaths of women in the year after childbirth are from suicide.

Help is most effective when developed in the context of a policy framework that includes all health services and statutory and voluntary agencies. Cooperation is vital.[13]

A model for how a project can be run is provided in the city of Leeds. A multi-agency approach involves the West Yorkshire Police and trains medical students, senior house officers, obstetricians, gynaecologists, the neonatal team, trainee general practitioners, midwives, health visitors, nursing students, healthcare assistants, hospital administrators, and accident and emergency staff. They have input into child protection courses, and focus especially on the needs of black women, disabled women, and women who are marginalised for any reason. The workers in this project emphasise the huge need for pre-registration teaching of all health professionals. Although this is happening in Leeds, it is not yet national policy.

Nurses and midwives are often concerned that to ask questions about abuse will alienate and anger women. Yes, some are shocked by questions they did not expect and that they consider intrusive. Yet a study in Sweden of pregnant women's responses to being asked by their midwives whether they had experienced any violence revealed that 80% found the question acceptable, 17% were in two minds on the subject, and only 3% said it was unacceptable.[14]

The Royal College of Midwives suggests that questions that invite a woman to talk about violence can be general, such as 'Is everything all right at home?', or more specific, such as, 'Some women tell me that their partners hit them. Has that happened to you?', 'I notice you have some bruising. Did anyone at home do that to you?', 'Are you frightened of anyone at home?', 'Is anyone hurting you at home?', 'Does your partner break things that belong to you?'. These more specific questions are highly intrusive and probing and could only ever enable a woman to open up when an atmosphere of trust and mutuality has been created. Midwives and other health professionals represent powerful institutions. Women know this. When confronted with such a display of power a pregnant woman may feel even more isolated, helpless and trapped. For any conversation to be effective, women obviously need to be able to talk to their midwives without a partner or other family member present. Yet under one-half of all maternity hospitals offer women any appointments without their partners.[6]

In the course of a training scheme for midwives it was discovered that, although there was already a question about violence on the antenatal care booking form, midwives sometimes omitted the question, asked it but did so in the presence of the woman's partner, or had no idea what to do if the woman said she was being abused.

Midwives are understandably reluctant to quiz women and invade their privacy. Following a conference to announce government plans for health workers to question pregnant women, a columnist in the *Sunday Times* published a tirade about 'this monstrous new initiative', said she did not accept the statistics, and that it amounted to 'a license to cross-question and monitor every single pregnant woman in the country. That is, without exaggeration, an outrage and a very typically New Labour collectivist outrage'.[15] Such strongly felt objections need to be confronted.

Abused women have a right to confidentiality, and their autonomy must be respected. They are most at risk if they decide to leave the relationship, and must not be put under pressure to do this.[16] A woman may be referred to a refuge, and needs to work out an 'exit plan' if she decides to leave home in a hurry, perhaps having a suitcase with clothes and other necessities, spare car keys, and essential documents for her and her children in a safe hiding place or with a neighbour. If she already has children, she should be told that if there is any chance that they could be harmed, confidentiality cannot be guaranteed. Women should be made aware of the help available through posters in toilets, booklets, and printed cards that give phone numbers of local and national Women's Aid, police community safety units, victim support, and social services – and these cards must be small enough to hide.

The needs of ethnic minority women have to be addressed with cultural awareness and sensitivity. Pregnant women from the Indian subcontinent are often accompanied to the clinic by a family member, usually a male partner or a young boy, to translate. Then it may be impossible to reveal abuse.

It may be important for caregivers to share their concerns with advocates from the minority groups involved, and perhaps help the woman get police protection, too.

A woman was forced into an arranged marriage at the age of 15 with a man who wanted to emigrate to the UK. He could not get a visa, and she returned home to the UK without him. Some years later she fell in love, got pregnant, and refused an abortion, although she was under heavy pressure from her family to have one, because of the disgrace of an illegitimate child for the family. Her midwives did all they could to help her, but then she told them that she had had a long talk with her mother and was out of danger. Everyone relaxed, glad that it was over and done with. At that point, a hired assassin killed her. Another pregnant woman, who left her husband because of his violence, which she disclosed during an antenatal visit, was offered support, but was murdered a few days after the baby's birth. Although all the relevant services were involved while she was pregnant, a complete breakdown in communication occurred once the baby had been born. In these cases midwives and social workers tried to help, but there was no continuity of care.

Ignorance, trivialisation of abuse, and failure of different agencies to collaborate with each other systematically and over time allows this violence to continue in a conspiracy of silence.

References

1. World Health Organisation 1997 Violence against women information pack: a priority health issue. Geneva: WHO

2. Mirrlees-Black C 1999 Domestic violence: findings from a new British Crime Survey self-completion questionnaire. London: Home Office

3. Mezey GC, Bewley S, Bacchus L, et al 2000 An exploration of the prevalence and effects of domestic violence in pregnancy. Swindon: Economics and Social Research Council

4. Lewis G (ed) 2001 Why mothers die 1997–99: Fifth report of the confidential enquiries into maternal deaths in the United Kingdom. London: RCOG Press

5. Women's Aid Federation of England 2001 Health and domestic violence survey 2000. London: Women's Aid Federation of England

6. Marchant S, Davidson LL, Garcia J, et al 2001 Addressing domestic violence through maternity services: policy and practice. Midwifery 17(3):164–270

7. Garcia J, Davidson LL 2002 Researching domestic violence and health. National Perinatal Epidemiology Unit. MIDRS Midwifery Digest 12(2):S25–S29

8. Ramsay J, Richardson J, Carter YH, et al 2002 Should health professionals screen women for domestic violence? Systematic review. BMJ 325(7359):314–318

9. Weldon F 2002 You ask the questions. Independent, 9 May

10. Hedin LW 2000 Postpartum, also a risk period for domestic violence. European Journal of Obstetrics, Gynecology and Reproductive Biology 89(1):41–45

11. Royal College of Obstetricians and Gynaecologists 1998 Why mothers die: confidential enquiries into maternal deaths in the UK, 5th report. London: RCOG Press

12. Women's Aid Federation of England 2001 Health and domestic violence survey 2000. London: Women's Aid Federation of England

13. Hepburn M, McCartney S 1997 Domestic violence and reproductive healthcare in Glasgow. In: Bewley S, Friend J, Mezey GC (eds) Violence against women. London: RCOG Press, p 233

14. Stenson K, Saarinen H, Heimer G, et al 2001 Women's attitudes to being asked about exposure to violence. Midwifery 17(1):1–10

15. Marrin M 2004 Have you stopped beating your pregnant wife yet? Sunday Times, 24 October, p 21

16. Bewley S, Gibb A 2001 Domestic abuse and pregnancy: writing policies and protocols. MIDIRS Midwifery Digest 11(2):183–187

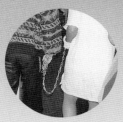

20
Mothers and babies behind bars

The number of women in British prisons has increased from 1800 a decade ago to over 4500 today. Many of them have drug problems and are mentally ill, or have committed minor offences, and a large proportion have not been convicted of anything, but are on remand awaiting trial.

In April 1995, after six male prisoners escaped from a prison and one woman absconded from an antenatal clinic and went home to see how her children were getting on, the Conservative Home Secretary, Michael Howard, enthusiastic about the American criminal justice system, ordered that all prisoners should be chained on journeys outside prison, including hospital visits.

In many American states prisoners have to wear metal shackles when in labour, until they have had an epidural to paralyse them from the waist down. In Arkansas, for example, women used to have one leg shackled to the hospital bed with an 18-inch chain, until the active second stage. There was a change of policy in 2004 and now these women are put under armed guard instead.

In Britain, pregnant women attending antenatal clinics and women in labour were shackled to two prison officers, one of whom might be a man, and the chains often remained on for most of the time they were in hospital, including during childbirth and when they were feeding their babies. Such shackling contravenes Britain's human rights obligations, and there is a strong case that it is illegal in both national and international law. The European Convention on Human Rights states that there must be no 'cruel, inhuman and degrading treatment' of prisoners, and the minimum standards set by the United Nations are that 'Chains should not be used.'

Birth chains

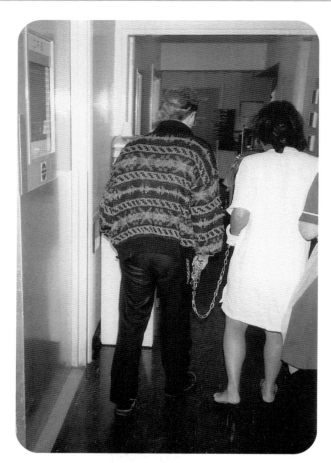

A prisoner who has just given birth in hospital, shackled to a prison officer
(Reproduced with permission of Beverley Lawrence Beech)

I briefed parliamentarians and conducted a media campaign to alert the public to what was happening and a group of us worked together to free women from their chains. A swift campaign focused on the single issue of getting women prisoners out of chains when in childbirth, and I rang colleagues in the Royal College of Midwives, the National Childbirth Trust (NCT), the Association for the Improvement of the Maternity Services and the Maternity Alliance, as well as the Howard League for Penal Reform and Women in Prison. We agreed that there was no time for lengthy committee meetings and that we must act immediately, taking responsibility as key individuals in our organisations, and aiming at speed and efficiency. These organisations had never worked together in quite this way before, but it seemed the right time to cooperate. I drafted a letter to the press which was published in the *Guardian* on 17 November 1995:[1]

> We should like to draw attention to a barbaric practice in the current treatment of pregnant women in prisons in England.
>
> In April last the Home Office issued an instruction that all women prisoners should be handcuffed to a prison officer when outside the prison. For many women this includes being shackled while attending for maternity appointments and during the birth of their babies. The implication is that if the shackles are

removed these women will immediately attempt to escape, even during labour, or that they will commit crimes of violence against the medical staff.

Latest statistics show that 56 women gave birth in outside hospitals whilst imprisoned during 1993/94. Despite denials from both the Prison Service and Home Office, the recent report from the Howard League for Penal Reform reveals that pregnant women are still kept shackled during antenatal care, labour and birth.

From many examples of which we know we cite one: a woman was shackled to two officers, one of whom was male, during her antenatal examination. The same woman subsequently was handcuffed and chained throughout a three-day stay in hospital, including when she used the lavatory. Her baby is due next month.

The majority of women prisoners have been convicted of poverty-related crimes, with only a tiny minority convicted of violent crime. Such treatment of pregnant women is barbaric. Pregnancy and birth are an intensely emotional and personal experience. This practice ensures that it is an inhumane process, which degrades the child-bearing woman and all those involved in her care.

We rightly criticise the abuse of women in some other cultures. We see this practice as a human rights issue which should be addressed immediately.

The letter was signed by: Mary Barnard, Chairman, NCT; Fiona Blake, Consultant Liaison Psychiatrist, John Radcliffe Hospital, Oxford; Caroline Flint, President, Royal College of Midwives; Meg Goodman, Health Policy Officer, Maternity Alliance; Sheila Kitzinger, Honorary Professor, Thames Valley University; Ann Oakley, Professor of Sociology and Social Policy, University of London; Lesley Page, Queen Charlotte's Professor of Midwifery; Gordon M. Stirrat, Professor of Obstetrics and Gynaecology, University of Bristol.

The Royal College of Obstetricians and Gynaecologists declined to sign because they said they were not prepared to get involved in 'human rights issues', although their President wrote to the Home Secretary expressing his concern about the practice of shackling. A *British Medical Journal* editorial stressed that 'doctors can object to seeing patients in shackles on the grounds that it is a degrading experience for both parties. Guidance on good practice from Britain's General Medical Council says that doctors must respect patients' privacy and dignity. It is not dignified for a patient to be shackled to a bed, or to be chained to a prison officer during a physical examination or treatment. Such physical restraints also ruin the trust and confidentiality between doctors and patients.'[2]

I drafted a statement, and together with the NCT, the Maternity Alliance and the Howard League, briefed researchers for the two opposition parties in the House of Commons, contacted individual parliamentarians in both Houses who had already spoken out on issues concerning women, health or the prison system, and prepared other briefing documentation. Parliamentary questions were asked and motions raised. I rang journalists with whom I had done work previously and said, 'I think I have a story for you.'

The media campaign was quick off the mark. The Government ministers responsible for the prison system protested that women were chained only if they were dangerous. TV producers wanted film evidence that women really were chained. Beverley Lawrence Beech of the Association for the Improvement of Maternity Services (AIMS) had on the previous day been a birth companion to a prisoner, Annette (sentenced to 2 years for stealing a purse), who had her baby in the Whittington Hospital. During part of labour, Annette was chained to two prison officers, one of whom was male. Beverley asked for a screen to be set up when Annette was in the second stage, but otherwise they watched vaginal examinations and other intimate procedures and, even after they were behind the screen, they could hear every sound. Beverley returned fitted with a hidden camera to record for Channel 4 News what happened postpartum. The result was stunning: TV news, which also made press headlines, editorials, cartoons, and chat shows and in-depth discussions on TV and radio. Over the next 2 weeks it was almost impossible to open a newspaper or switch on the TV or radio without encountering references to the issue.

On 24 January 1996 the Government announced a change in policy and practice. Ann Widdecombe, the Home Office Minister responsible for prisons, announced in the House of Commons: 'Female prisoners who are admitted to hospital to give birth will not have handcuffs or other physical restraints applied to them from the time they arrive at the hospital until the time they leave' and 'Restraints will not be applied at all during antenatal appointments.' We had done it! So far as policy is concerned. A sharply focused and rapidly executed campaign had been 100% successful. And 8 years later practice is different.

I also wrote about women being in chains during birth in the Blackwell Science journal, *Birth*.[3] Blackwell Science was threatened with a suit for libel. I declined to withdraw what I had written. The threat of litigation died down.

Based at a Manchester hospital, a new midwifery service was developed for prisoners in Styal 'to provide midwifery care which is woman centred, recognises and is sensitive to the needs of each individual woman with the emphasis on choice, continuity and control throughout the pregnancy continuum, at the same time ensuring accessibility of all services.'[4]

Community midwives also now go into Holloway Prison to give antenatal care there, and pregnant women visit hospital usually only for ultrasound scans. Staff shortages in the prison service are severe, so women miss appointments if two officers are not free to accompany them. It is a great advance, however, to have NHS midwives providing continuity of care and carer in Holloway.

Amnesty International recommends that 'Policies on the use of restraints should prohibit their use on pregnant women when they are being transported and when they are in hospital awaiting delivery' and on 'women who have just given birth'.[5]

But women are still shackled on their way to and from hospital. The chains are removed in the waiting room in most cases, except where the prisoner is estimated to be a security risk. This means, of course, that women are regularly shackled in early labour before they are admitted to hospital. They are still accompanied by two prison officers, one of whom may be a man, and remain under surveillance right through the birth, although the officers are behind a screen.

If the newborn baby is taken to the special care nursery, as many are to check that they have not been affected by any drugs taken by their mothers, the women are shackled again, and the cuffs are removed only when they visit their babies in the nursery.

The Birth Companions

Although it was a victory to release women from chains during labour and birth, a great deal remained to be done. I explored the possibility with NCT teachers in the area of Holloway Prison of setting up a doula scheme, to offer woman-to-woman support in late pregnancy, during birth and afterwards. Holloway is the largest women's prison in Europe. There was already an NCT antenatal teacher working in the prison and the breastfeeding counsellor became one of our doula group. We were fortunate to have help from Penny Simkin, who had trained well over a thousand doulas in the USA, and one noteworthy meeting was the day she spent with us at my house focusing on the skills needed for this work.

The prison doulas are now renamed Birth Companions. They help women who want to do so to handle birth physiologically by moving around, breathing and being massaged, and to breastfeed. They also support a woman who opts for an epidural or is having a caesarean section. They give unconditional friendship and simple woman-to-woman help in pregnancy, during childbirth, and in the days afterwards.

One grandmother told me:

> When I arrived at the hospital I was surprised to see a woman comforting and cherishing my daughter. She not only stayed for the birth but she and another 'birth sister' helped with the care of mother and baby throughout their time in hospital. They are the most selfless people I have ever met.

Describing her experience of birth, a prisoner wrote:

> I was made to feel at ease and even though in a lot of pain I was conscious of her always being there. I had more faith and trust in my birthing partner than anyone else ... You guys have rebuilt my trust and faith in human nature.

The work the Birth Companions are pioneering is vitally important. But this is not enough.

In Holloway, 27% of women are single mothers, over half of these had their first child when they were teenagers, and 34% are black. Many have been sexually abused. Some are self-harming. Some are mentally ill. Few have been convicted of violent crimes. It is more likely that they are in prison for drug-related offences, petty theft or benefit fraud. Overall, 33% are first time offenders. But many have not been convicted of any offence – 27% are on remand. These remand prisoners are incarcerated on average for 110 days.

The Prison Reform Trust reports:

> *Two-thirds of women show symptoms of at least one neurotic disorder, such as depression, anxiety and phobias. More than half are suffering from a personality disorder. Among the general population less than a fifth of women suffer from these disorders. Half of the women in prison are on prescribed medication such as anti-depressants or anti-psychotic medicine and there is evidence that the use of medication increases whilst in custody. Of all the women who are sent to prison, 37% say they have attempted suicide at some time in their life.*[6]

Taking babies from their mothers

A woman in Holloway is not sure until the last 5 or 6 weeks of pregnancy whether she will be allowed to keep her baby. She cannot prepare emotionally for the time following birth or allow herself to bond with her baby. Women sometimes tell their families: 'Don't buy any clothes for the baby.' They are in an emotional limbo. This is because towards the end of pregnancy a board meeting is held to decide whether the woman will be admitted to the Mother and Baby Unit. She may be considered unsuitable because she talks back to prison officers, gets into conflict with other prisoners, or does not obey orders.

The Holloway Prison Board sits about 6 weeks before the baby is due. It consists of someone at the grade of a prison governor, a prison officer, a prison doctor, a probation officer and a social worker. There is no psychiatrist, no midwife and no psychotherapist.

A 24-year-old psychology student, whom I shall call 'Jane', in prison on a 5-year sentence for slashing a friend's face with a craft knife in an argument over a man – her first offence – was told that her baby would be taken away at birth. She decided to challenge the decision. I learned about this soon after the Holloway board meeting, obtained the minutes of the meeting from the solicitor, contacted the woman's mother and the woman herself, and determined to fight this to the end. I rang the head of the psychology department at the university where Jane was studying, who believed that the behaviour was 'totally out of character' and that 'she was drowning in personal problems'. He was right. She was in an abusive relationship with a man who was beating her up.

A decision of the Holloway Board had never been challenged before. This Board had no doctor on it, which it should have had, and accusations were unsubstantiated. For the most part they were petty. The woman was 'disruptive'; she took a carton of milk that was not hers; she was accused of throwing it at an officer, who later remembered that this had been another prisoner 2 weeks before; she had made 'snide remarks' to a woman who was reduced to tears; she picked quarrels and bullied other prisoners; she did not get up in the morning. This occurred when she was told that her AFP (α-fetoprotein) level suggested she had a Down's syndrome baby, and an amniocentesis revealed that the baby had an extra chromosome. She did not seem to be looking forward to being a mother and was not excited about the baby, one Board member complained, and the implication was that for this reason the baby should be removed from her. Another, a health visitor, said that to care for a baby you need to be able to cooperate with everyone. Board members and prison officers need education to understand the combined stresses of imprisonment, pregnancy and screening procedures. Even some from outside the prison appear to have been institutionalised and to have accepted the prison culture.

Jane's solicitors asked me to be an expert witness, but I proposed that John Davis, Emeritus Professor of Paediatrics at Cambridge University, should do this. With a statement from him they went to the Crown Court and were granted leave to appeal. I was concerned that there had been no independent psychological assessment. I asked Dr Suzie Orbach if she would do one free of charge and she did so immediately. She pointed out in her report that Jane was suffering from both shock and depression. I also thought it important to have a senior barrister, but the solicitors did not know if Legal Aid would pay for this. In fact, they did get Legal Aid for a specialist in human rights.

I rang journalists and there was lively interest. Meanwhile Jane had given birth on the day that the first attempt at an appeal was turned down. She learned that the case had failed just after she delivered her baby daughter. 'After she was born, I couldn't sleep. I just lay looking at her all night. It is difficult with two prison officers sitting watching you in a small room day and night. I can't eat. Now, as the time comes when they will take her from me, I can't even look at her properly because I don't want to get too attached. Her tiny hands – they're usually closed up in tight little fists. But when I'm breastfeeding her I put a finger in her hand and she wraps her hand round it … When I'm breastfeeding her she stares up at me, and she knows me!' Then she wept uncontrollably. When at last she could speak again, she went on: 'I don't know whether I dare cuddle her. I long to pick her up and to hold her. But they are going to take my baby away from me and I don't know what to do. One of the prison governors came yesterday with someone else from the prison I think, but she didn't introduce us. She was so cold. She just walked in and told me the social services would come for the baby on Friday. I thought I had more time, that they wouldn't take the baby until an appeal in the High Court, but she said "No". They were taking her, She just strode in and said that, and she didn't even look at the baby'. Jane told me, 'If they take my baby away from me they might as well kill me'. The hospital agreed to keep Jane with her baby until the verdict of the Court was announced. Jane gave me permission to let a journalist with the *Independent* newspaper have the number of the phone at her bedside. As far as the prison officers were concerned she was talking to a friend. I kept in close touch with the press and TV and Frances Crook of the

Howard League threw her energy and her knowledge of the prison system into the campaign. The Maternity Alliance also became involved and, because Jane was breastfeeding her baby, I solicited help from breastfeeding organisations. On the day of the Crown Court appeal, mothers, fathers and babies from these organisations turned up outside with big notices saying: 'Remember the child'.

Counsel for Jane focused on the rights of the child. Counsel for Holloway asked for more time to prepare his case. When one of the three judges asked, 'Are you going to tear this baby from her mother's breast?' those of us who were determined to keep mother and baby together felt the first flush of success. The judges asked the Counsel for Holloway whether, if he was given the week for which he asked, he could assure the Court that mother and baby would be kept together during that time.

The barrister wheeled round and asked the representatives of Holloway whether that could be arranged. There was an awkward pause. He turned back, with obvious embarrassment, 'No, my Lord'. The judges' eyebrows shot up into their wigs. One said, 'You do surprise me!' Another, 'You can't? Goodness me!' They allowed him the weekend to get his act together, but insisted that mother and baby were not separated.

Over that weekend the solicitors for Holloway contacted Jane's solicitors to try and arrange a settlement. When the Court assembled it was agreed that the Board should sit again. It was stipulated that the Board consist of different people, be chaired by someone from outside the prison, and none of the previous anecdotes about her behaviour should be considered, because none had been proved.

This case created a practical precedent. The judges ruled that, in future, primary consideration must be given to the rights of the child. Every prison must honour the rules of the European Human Rights Convention and the United Nations Convention on the Rights of the Child. Holloway had neglected to comply with prison service regulations and, in future, the Board should be properly constituted, the correct protocol observed, and a prisoner should have the right to a legal representative.

The Governor of Holloway resigned the day after the Crown Court appeal. Richard Tilt, then Director of the Prison Service, announced a review of principles, policies and procedures for mothers and babies and the setting up of a working group to include professionals from health, social and probation services and relevant interest groups.

Holloway was unwilling to have Jane back and she was admitted to the Mother and Baby Unit at Styal prison. She resumed her psychology studies in prison and kept her baby with her. I worked with the solicitor to appeal against her sentence when her daughter was approaching 18 months, the time when the child would have been taken from her. We won the appeal and Jane was released on bail immediately.

Prison is not the right place

More than one-third of all women in prison have been convicted for minor infringements of the law, and for what are essentially crimes of poverty. A large proportion are foreign nationals who have been caught bringing drugs into the country.

On the Holloway special maternity wing women often share cells, and a prisoner who has just had a miscarriage or abortion may be locked up with a pregnant woman. There is little to do except lie in bed, and staff shortages result in women often being locked in for all but an hour a day. Many women are disturbed, or become disturbed, in prison, and self-harm with razor blades is common. The punishment for this is almost invariably further cell confinement. Officers receive no training in the special needs of women who cut themselves or try to commit suicide. Physical conditions are bad, and inspectors have reported cells infested with rats and cockroaches, and used tampons and waste food thrown through windows because there was nowhere else to dispose of them. In the same year that Michael Howard introduced his 'get tough' policy, the Chief Inspector of Prisons walked out of a snap inspection in protest at 'overzealous security, prisoners being locked up in their cells for 23 hours a day, poor healthcare, bullying, low staff morale, inadequate education and activities, and very dirty conditions'.[7]

I feel strongly that our commitment to help childbearing women must extend to speaking out for the most vulnerable women in our society, and that it is not acceptable for birth organisations to restrict their work to those who are most privileged. It is not that we do this deliberately, of course, but it is so much easier to reach out to and communicate with women who form part of our usual social networks. Women in prison include the poorest, the least educated, those who have suffered violence and who have been sexually abused, the mentally ill, and women for whom it is most difficult to cope with the stresses of incarceration. Pregnancy can be an opportunity for learning, development, change and maturation and for commitment to a new life. An opportunity is being lost for rehabilitation, for giving emotional support, helping women to understand the relationships in which they are caught up, and planning ahead for after the baby's birth.

Many issues remain to be addressed, not least whether pregnant women and women with young children should be incarcerated at all. In a debate in the House of Lords, Lord Dholakia said: 'Ultimately, there should be a situation where only in exceptional circumstances, and for very serious matters, women should receive custodial sentences. Let us enshrine that in our sentencing guidelines. With women, we are not just sentencing an individual, we are sentencing the whole family'.[8]

The effects of separation on children

At least 61% of women in British prisons are mothers of children under the age of 18, and nearly one-third of these children are less than 5 years old, and the mother is the sole carer. Because women fear their children will be taken into care by the Social Services, some keep it secret that they have children. Every year approximately 17,700 children are separated from their imprisoned mothers. Half of all the babies who are being cared for by other people because their mothers are in prison are shifted between two and four different homes before their first birthday.[9]

When a woman is released from prison she may face the challenge of building a relationship with a child who is emotionally disturbed, both because he or she has been separated from her during the first year, and also because the child has been switched between different caregivers. It is vital for an infant to form a strong attachment to one person during those 12 months.[10] All other attachments grow from that first love affair. From it develops a sense of security and trust and the capacity for love and self-esteem.[11] A child denied this is at risk of becoming an adult unable to have satisfying relationships and who is antisocial and emotionally disturbed.

Whenever a baby is taken away from its mother we punish the baby as well as the mother. Mothers and babies belong together. Separation is an emotional mutilation for both of them. Babies are the most vulnerable members of society. To penalise them for a crime the mother has committed is an abuse of adult power. The prison system could not be better designed to turn out young people who are bitter, and at risk of further damaging themselves and hitting out against society. And for mothers it is another form of institutionalised violence against women.

Imprisonment of a mother punishes older children, too. When a woman is sentenced, for 85% of children it is the first time they have been separated from their mother for more than a day or so.[9] Only 3% of women prisoners have a child with them in prison. Until recently there have been only 64 places in Mother and Baby Units, although there are plans (2004) for new units to accommodate around 120 mothers with their children. (Clearly, there is no intention to provide an alternative system to prison.) The baby is taken from them at 9 months of age if they are in Holloway and at 18 months, or earlier, if they are in a prison such at Styal, where there is a Mother and Baby Unit that accepts children up to that age. So children are farmed out. Usually granny has to take over or they go into care.

When mothers in prison are asked about children who are not with them almost half say that they are worried about problems with their behaviour that have developed since their imprisonment. This is especially the case when Social Services place the children in foster care and families are split up. Siblings are separated for the first time in their lives. They, too, may get shifted from one caregiver to another.

The most likely consequence is that the child becomes withdrawn and depressed. Caddel and Crisp[9] reveal that one in four such children have difficulties sleeping or become physically ill. Some start bed-wetting. It is sometimes very difficult for those caring for these children to understand and help them through their grieving. The Jamaican grandmother of one 6 year old rang me regularly because she could not cope with the little girl's depression. She took her to a child psychiatrist. But what the child really needed was her mother. After a series of psychiatric reports and representations by her solicitors and others, this mother, with her baby born while she was in prison, was released on bail. But the process of getting them together took a long time. I suspect that has had a profound effect on this child's developing personality.

Because prisons are often a long distance from where families live, visiting is difficult. In this way society punishes the whole family. Amnesty International states: 'Maintaining close relationships with their children provides a powerful incentive for prisoners to participate in and benefit from rehabilitative programs; and maintaining strong family ties during imprisonment decreases recidivism'.[12]

Women in prison and drugs

In the 1990s many female Nigerian 'mules' were convicted of carrying drugs into the UK. Their children were in Nigeria and they thought they were making a trip to Britain that would last several days and then would be home. Instead they found themselves in prison with anything up to a 10-year sentence. Now many Nigerian women are refusing to be drug runners. Caribbean women come in their place. One in 16 women prisoners is a Jamaican convicted of smuggling cocaine or other drugs. Many have no previous convictions. Drug gangs target hospitals in Jamaica to pick up poor women who need to raise money for medical treatment. These prisoners lose all contact with their children apart from a phone call every 4 weeks or so. They cannot afford to phone more often than that.

In the USA, too, increasing numbers of women are imprisoned for drug offences: 'Without any fanfare "the war on drugs" has become a war on women. This has clearly contributed to the explosion in the women's prison population'.[12]

Anticipatory grieving/anticipatory freezing

Forced separation from her baby is one of the most traumatic life events that a woman can experience. We have seen that if a woman is pregnant when she is imprisoned she faces the terrible uncertainty of not knowing whether she can keep her baby. She feels in limbo. She may switch off emotionally from the pregnancy or enter a state of anticipatory grieving. The bonding process, far from being an instant glue that attaches a mother and baby after birth, begins in pregnancy. When a woman dare not bond she may screen out fetal movements and regard her baby simply as an awkward bump or, at worst, a kind of cancer. Then, when the baby is born, she tries to stay as detached as possible.

In the USA there is usually no question of a mother keeping her baby, and it is removed at birth. The Reverend Cathy Arends, who is also a psychiatric nurse, is a chaplain at the Louisiana Correctional Institute for Women. She has managed to get women out of chains in childbirth, but only if they have an epidural. She sees women weekly through pregnancy, one-to-one and privately, and is a companion to them during the birth. She tried to start a newborn nursery, but the Department of Correction cancelled the programme because of 'fear of a hostage situation', and she is trying to establish an alternative sentencing facility for pregnant, non-violent, first-time offenders, but without success.

This prison has a 'no tears policy'. Any inmate who is observed crying or who writes a letter home sharing her grief, is put in lock-down for 90 days, under suicide watch. This adds 90 days to her sentence for 'bad behaviour'. Once a week, when prisoners visit Cathy, they are able to weep: 'Often they come in, close the door, cry for 10–15 minutes, give me a hug and leave. That time will sustain them till the next visit'.

In 1997 in Britain, Roisin McAlisky, daughter of the Irish MP Bernadette Devlin, and a politics graduate at the time, was arrested on suspicion of terrorism and imprisoned in Holloway. She was in early pregnancy. The Home Secretary, Jack Straw, held her on remand in custody pending her extradition to be tried in Germany, where she was accused of blowing up a car on a British Army base. Roisin denied the charge. The case against her was thin. During the period when she was alleged to have been planning the attack she was employed by the Irish World organisation, which provides training places for the disabled, the long-term unemployed and ex-offenders from both communities. So, when I spoke to her, I did not feel I was communicating with a likely terrorist. But that is beside the point. Here was a woman passing through a great transition in her life and bringing a baby into the world. She was held in isolation from other prisoners. She was let out of her small cell for 1 hour out of the 24 – if she was lucky. The light was kept on day and night. Reading material was taken away at 8 p.m. and not returned until the morning.

Working with her solicitor, Gareth Peirce, a specialist on issues of human rights, I was able to find expert witnesses – a Professor of Paediatrics, a Professor of Midwifery and a consultant obstetrician – to examine her health and obtain more humane care. Professor John Davis, Professor of Paediatrics at Cambridge, said: 'If you asked "What is the ideal place for a baby to be born into?" this is the exact opposite. No human being should come into the world in these circumstances'. As soon as her baby daughter was born, I enlisted the help of Channi Kumar, Professor of Psychiatry at the Maudsley Hospital, who testified that she was at risk of postpartum depression. He agreed to admit her to the Maudsley Psychiatric Mother and Baby Unit, where she stayed until her baby was 10 months old and, following a vigorous campaign to release her, the Home Secretary decided not to extradite her, and she was freed.

Roisin has written for me an in-depth, retrospective analysis of the emotional experience of being imprisoned in pregnancy and not knowing whether she could keep her baby. Other mothers may not all feel as she did. But her narrative has lessons for all those concerned with the treatment of pregnant prisoners.

In the highly artificial and overcrowded conditions of prison women are in constant fear of violence. It is similar to the condition of animals caged in a zoo. Zuckerman studied primates living in zoo conditions and described how they were aggressive much of the time. He considered this an inherent characteristic. However, when the same primates were studied in their natural habitat, no similar level of aggression was observed. The hostility and conflict was a result of the conditions in which they were imprisoned. When human beings are denied any control over how they live and are crowded together, aggression may be one way in which they try to assert identity.

Prisoners may experience sensory alienation from their bodies as a way of resisting physical shackling and the invasion of body boundaries if they are strip-searched, which involves physical exposure, inherent threat and humiliation. Roisin wrote to me: 'As I was undergoing strip-searching, my body was not something that I wished to focus on or think about. As a form of defence I deliberately did not consider my physical self'.

No full-length mirrors are allowed in prison, since these could be broken and used as weapons or for self-harm. So there is an absence of reflected image. Roisin wrote: 'One restriction that I now believe as having had the most detrimental effect on me was the fact that my isolation not only removed me from other people, for conversation, for example, but that I had no contact with pregnant women. There were not even any mirrors. I never saw the size I was until 3 days before giving birth, and I lost connection with my body. I knew I was pregnant, I knew I was going to become a mother. I did know that carrying a baby was making me fat. I forgot what fat looked like. I forgot me. Yes, I saw maternity magazines. Yes, I saw pregnant women from afar and caught side-long looks at them waddling around corridors. I didn't get to see them move, try to sit, try to eat when the table is too far away because of the bump. So to my mind I didn't get to see me do those things either'. When she saw herself in a full-length mirror during a hospital visit she fainted.

Seven years later she wrote to me: 'Now, if I'm honest, I find it hard to watch those things. I don't do the pregnancy conversation. I'm quite oblivious to bumps. I have no connection to bumps. I never had'.

There is deprivation and distortion of sensory experience of the environment. This is how Roisin described it: 'There is no smell, except for cleaner and there is no colour, except for pale. There is no view and it's never dark and it's never light. It's all fluorescent. And the noises are either echoes or thuds, until you learn not to hear them at all. I simply couldn't breathe, or see, or hear, or feel in that place. What I didn't know at that point was all the things I'd missed in jail. Being touched – by anyone who isn't holding a mirror to look in those awkward out of the way bodily places'.

In pregnancy a woman perceives her baby both as self and as other. The alternative to sensory deadening and withdrawal from the baby is to be destroyed in another way. A pregnant woman who has not detached herself from her body like this, who has not succeeded in anaesthetising herself against pain, and who has bonded to her unborn baby, faces the threat of separation as if it were to be torn in two. Roisin repressed physical sensations during pregnancy. She wrote: 'I was totally unprepared for the realisation of the separation during birth. I am not sure which came first, the fear of my loss or the relief of her safety. Separation is something I had to consider. I don't view this as any choice that I was given. Choice implies that there exists some voluntary input. The phrase "I have no choice" should be the property only of those who have lived through no choice. I really didn't know until I heard her first scream what separation meant. It is all hypothetical until that first scream. To separate or not to separate from your baby? What baby? You haven't had it yet! Most ridiculous, illogical, insulting questions asked by men in suits and women in chains. And when you can't answer it, you fail, and when you do answer it, you fail, and before the baby is even born you are a failure. You are a failure as a mother. One hell of a start. Or a finish. I have no idea how mothers who have to give their babies up in jail get them back. Physically, maybe. Emotionally, I doubt it'.

To be admitted to the Mother and Baby Unit the prisoner must have been successfully institutionalised. She must be free of drugs, obedient and submissive. Roisin was never admitted to the Mother and Baby Unit, but I discussed with her ways in which women might adjust well to that environment and be emotionally better grounded than outside in the community. She commented: 'Swapping a high rise tower block and debt to the loan shark, the drug dealer, the neighbour, for a high rise prison block and just to get to a nameless, faceless society that never really liked you anyway. To some people one concrete cage can be more comfortable than another'.

A ticket to motherhood

Will they be good mothers? No one can predict how a woman is going to be as a mother. The most awkward, the most irresponsible, young woman has the potential to turn into a wonderful mother. If you have children, think back to how you were before the birth of your first baby. If you had been forced to take an exam in motherhood, if you had been assessed by experts, would you have passed or failed? When, after a long struggle, Jane's case went to the Crown Court, a judge raised this point. The barrister representing Holloway Prison had stated that the Board which had made the decision that Jane should not be accepted into the Mother and Baby Unit there came to this conclusion because she was a difficult and disruptive prisoner. The Judge commented that he was not sure that if anyone had examined him as a young man he would ever have been considered suitable for fatherhood.

When a woman has behaved in a socially irresponsible way, punitive action may push her further into irresponsibility. If she is pregnant or has a young child, there is an opportunity to develop a sense of responsibility, increased emotional awareness and insight into human behaviour. But, to nurture her baby, a woman needs to be nurtured *herself*. It is not enough to give her lessons in child care. I talked to the woman who runs parentcraft classes in one of the prisons with a Mother and Baby Unit. She explained to me that the prisoners had 'theory' in the morning and did knitting in the afternoon. She is not very hopeful about the effects of the work she is doing. Neither am I.

As I read the minutes of the prison board meetings, making the decision to separate a baby from its mother, I am struck by the psychological limitations of their understanding. Some are not really minutes at all. They consist of gossip, innuendo, assumptions, accusations that a prisoner is 'disruptive' or 'argumentative' – and an almost complete lack of evidence. Until recently, the prisoner was given no information and was denied legal representation. In future, according to the Response and Action Plans in the report of a Review of Principles, Policies and Procedures on Mothers and Babies/Children in Prison,[13] the prisoner will be told of what she is accused, and allowed to speak for herself.

Prison and the National Health Service

Following exposure in the press and on radio and TV about the way pregnant women were treated, the situation improved in both Holloway and Styal. But the service is fragmented. Each prison seems to be a world to itself. The advances seen in Holloway since the publicity that surrounded Jane's Crown Court hearing in 1998 have not been matched in some other prisons. The Prison Service is providing new Mother and Baby units, services which support family ties, the appointment of a national coordinator for Mother and Baby Units, and for the first time it plans to train staff.

Many women in prison have been abused and are self-harming. They slash their arms and legs with razor blades, often after many years of being abused as children. Prison officers rarely distinguish between self-harm and suicide risk. The standard response is 'She's trying to draw attention to herself', and the woman is locked in a cell in which there is nothing with which she can cut or hurt herself. A prisoner in Holloway went into labour in a cell and told me that on her way to the ambulance she had to walk past the body of a young woman who cut her wrists and bled to death in a nearby cell. These women may simply feel despair or have a boiling anger inside them that they cannot control. Their experience of imprisonment compounds and exacerbates previous emotional trauma. Many have been beaten up and raped by the men in their lives. They hate themselves.

The late Channi Kumar, Professor of Perinatal Psychiatry at the Maudsley Hospital, told me: 'We need something to meet their emotional needs better than anything that can be provided in the prison setting. We need this not only for the mother's sake, but for the baby's, too'. Since 1964, the Royal College of Physicians has argued that the National Health Service (NHS) should take over the care of sick prisoners, and for more than 20 years the Royal College of Psychiatrists has urged that their members should care for the many prisoners who are mentally ill. An editorial in the *BMJ* in the 1980s urged the provision of mental health services in prisons: 'Prison is the main sewer of British society'.[14]

In 1999, the Editor of the *BMJ* again addressed the issue: 'Many of those who have watched the excruciating long and slow minuet between the prison service and the NHS will think that the final step of the NHS taking full responsibility must and should come soon ... Prison medicine is out of date with the very "medicalised model of care", focusing on illness not health and with little attention to prevention, guidelines, multidisciplinary audit, continuing professional development, or information ... Although some nursing staff do remarkable work in difficult conditions, many are security officers first and nurses second; and they have primitive training ... Prisons in England and Wales are overcrowded, insanitary, and dangerous and there is a very high prevalence of mental health problems and substance abuse among prisoners'.[15]

A report by HM Prisons Inspectorate into the care of the mentally ill revealed that, compared with 0.4% of the general population, 14% of female prisoners were suffering from psychosis – a rate twice as high as that for sentenced men – and that compared with 11% in the general population, 64% of women on remand had symptoms of depression. But not a single prison doctor was fully psychiatrically qualified and most nurses had no mental health training. The report concluded: 'The quality of service for mentally ill prisoners fell below the standards in the NHS. Patients' lives were unacceptably restricted and therapy limited. It is easy to be sucked into and overwhelmed by the ethos and practices of a powerful institution. The present policy of dividing inpatient care of mentally disordered prisoners between the prison service and the NHS needs reconsideration'.[16] A former Chief Inspector of Prisons, Sir David Ramsbotham, also recommended that the NHS take over prison healthcare. The Prison Service resisted this for years.

Coordination between mental health and midwifery services and the prison authorities is generally poor. It can be difficult to get to psychiatric appointments. In Holloway, mentally ill prisoners rarely have access to nursing staff at night, and nurses do not carry room keys. In an emergency the key and the staff member must be brought from the main prison, which takes at least 10 minutes. There is no midwife for pregnant women resident in the prison and they become very anxious that they may start labour at night, locked in their rooms. This was the case with a woman whose baby was subsequently born in a locked cell and died before she reached hospital. She had not been convicted. She was on remand.

The need for change

It is not enough to tinker with conditions inside prisons. Sentencing practice needs to change, too. When sentence is passed, there are often 'invisible' children. Whoever passes the sentence may not realise that children are involved, ignores their existence, or does not know that a woman is pregnant. Sometimes it is worse than that. A child may be perceived by a judge as a doll that can be taken away to punish a girl. A 17-year-old girl convicted of being a lookout for a friend who stole three shirts from Marks and Spencer's was sentenced to imprisonment until 2 weeks after her baby was due. The judge announced that the baby would be taken away from her in order to punish her.

It is time for radical reform. These women and babies should not be in prison at all. The United Nations recommends: 'The use of imprisonment for certain categories of offenders, such as pregnant women or mothers with infants or small children, should be restricted and a special effort made to avoid the use of imprisonment as a sanction for these categories'.[17]

I believe that we should explore the setting up of small 'family' hostels or cottage communities within 50 miles of a woman's home. Some prison officers look forward to running community-based units like this. They hoped that they would result from the inquiry into Principles, Policies and Procedures on Mothers and Babies.[13] Even so, they would need a lot of help to do this effectively. They may not necessarily be the right people. We should not assume that prison officers are ideal for this responsible task. It looks as if we are not going to get those new units anyway. The 1999 inquiry urged the Prison Service to explore with the Probation Service the potential for providing mother and baby facilities in hostel accommodation in the community. The response from the Prison Service stated baldly: 'A mixed facility is not feasible either legally or practically'.[13] Meanwhile, in Germany, women with children are held in houses under curfew in units outside the prison gates.

A cosmetic operation is not the answer. It is no solution to paint prison walls pink, hang up mobiles and load children with toys. It is not enough to bring yet more experts in to advise, to set up yet more committees, to ponder ways out of this degrading and abusive system.

We need to work out, at top political level, how our society can provide a positive environment for pregnancy, birth and motherhood for *everyone*. That is the challenge. Anne Owers, the Chief Inspector of Prisons, says: 'It is particularly the marginalised who need the protection of human rights. By definition prisons are closed environments. They operate outside the normal controls and processes of society; and it is often the case that society as a whole is less than interested about what happens behind their walls. We do not talk of "our prisons" as we talk of "our" schools and hospitals; politicians rarely feel the need to promise more prison officers, as they do more police or more doctors and teachers. Because they are out of sight and out of mind, prisons need to have a light shone on them, so that society as a whole can know what is being done in its name'.[18] Sentencing policies need to have a radical overhaul. In a debate in the House of Lords, Baroness Stern suggested that 'the remit of the Department of Health prison health service should be extended so that there is a role alongside the police when charging, the prosecution when prosecuting, and the Court when sentencing to say, "This is a health problem, not a crime problem. We must deal with it another way".[19]

The NHS took over healthcare in prisons in 2004. This can have a special impact on the well-being of mothers and babies, achieve health promotion for some of the most deprived members of society, and a positive effect on public health where needs are most acute.

We have seen that many pregnant women in prison have experienced sexual abuse and other forms of violence. They have often been in care as children, rates of literacy are low, and they have used drugs. One-to-one midwifery and continuity of care is vital for these women through pregnancy, birth and after. When one prisoner was discharged from hospital to Holloway shortly after she delivered her stillborn baby, she committed suicide. There was no continuity of care. Every pregnant prisoner needs a skilled confiding friend who can help her grow into motherhood, see herself and her relationships with fresh eyes and accept responsibility for a new life. This is a challenging role for a midwife. She needs to listen non-judgementally to a woman's anxieties and fears, support her in understanding and taking pride in her body as she goes through a major life transition, and enable her to feel valued, develop self-confidence, and be able to express love. Not only midwives, but everyone in the health service, can contribute to good outcomes for these women who have been battered by life.

A vital aspect of this work should be discussion groups for prison staff, especially officers in day-to-day contact with pregnant women and new mothers. Many have entered the prison service with high hopes, but do not have the training to understand the psychological aspects of being pregnant in prison and not knowing whether you can keep your baby until around 6 weeks before it is due.

When a mother and baby are together there is the option of breastfeeding. Prison officers tend to bring the attitude to baby feeding that they adopted with their own children. They can benefit from special training about how to give positive support for breastfeeding, and midwives are ideally placed to do this.

Women are still transferred to and from hospital in chains. The rule is that when 'treatment' begins the chains should be removed. A midwife can simply tell prison officers to unlock the chains as soon as a woman arrives at the hospital. She is now her patient. The practice of keeping women in pre-labour or early labour in a side-room in chains cannot be condoned.

The newborn baby is often taken to the special care nursery. When this happens the chains are put on again. Staff can insist that women are not in chains.

When NHS staff are working inside the prison, too, prisoners are entitled to the same quality of care and, wherever possible, the same choices as women in the community. It is easy for health staff to become institutionalised by the prison system and to take their lead from prison officers. They need to be confident, outgoing, and to focus on the health needs, both physical and psychological, of the women in their care.

I believe that we should work towards a Charter for the Health of Women Prisoners with standards of practice which NHS workers are proud to make a reality.

Ethics and opportunities

In Nazi Germany ordinary citizens protested that they knew nothing of what was going on in concentration camps. Today, it is easy to remain ignorant of conditions in prisons, as well as in detention centres for asylum seekers. I believe that any commitment to help childbearing women must extend to speaking out for the most vulnerable and voiceless women in our own society. Pregnancy can be an opportunity for development and change, a time when women experience nurturing, and when they can go on to take responsibility for a new life. It is an opportunity that must not be missed.

Still in 2005 a woman is not allowed to be legally represented at the Holloway board meeting. She may not know until a couple of weeks before the birth, or sometimes after she has given birth, if her baby will be taken away. That hangs on the judgement of the prison social worker. When a woman has a short sentence a newborn baby may be taken from its mother, who is unable to get to know or breastfeed her baby, only to be returned a few weeks later at the end of her sentence.

References

1. Kitzinger S, Barnard M, Blake F, et al 1995 Letter to the editor. Guardian, 17 November, p 10

2. Dillner L 1996 Shackling prisoners in hospital [editorial]. BMJ 312(7025):200

3. Kitzinger S 1994 Letter from England: prison babies. Birth 21(3):170–171

4. Scott L 1997 Report on the provision of maternity services for prisoners who are pregnant undergoing a custodial sentence within HM Prison Styal. South Manchester University Hospitals NHS Trust, January

5. Amnesty International 1999 Not part of my sentence: violations of the human rights of women in custody. Available at: http://web.amnesty.org/library/index/ENGAMR510191999 (accessed November 2004)

6. Prison Reform Trust 2004 Fact file. In: Lacking conviction. London: Prison Reform Trust, p 11 [Citing statistics from: O'Brien M, et al 1998 Psychiatric mortality among women prisoners in England and Wales. London: Office for National Statistics]

7. Ford R, Tendler S, King G 1995 Jail walkout by horrified inspectors: conditions at Holloway condemned. Times, 19 December, p 1

8. Lord Dholakia 2004 Debate on women in prison. Hansard, House of Lords, 28 October, column 1448

9. Caddel D, Crisp D 1997 Imprisoned women and mothers. Research study 162. London: Home Office Research and Statistics Directorate

10. Klaus MH, Kennell JH, Klaus PH 1996 Bonding – building the foundations of secure attachment and independence. London: Cedar

11. Winnicott DW 1988 Babies and their mothers, 2nd edn. New York: Addison Wesley

12. Bloom B, Chesney Lind M, Owen B 1994 Women in Californian prisons: hidden victims of the war on drugs. San Francisco: Center on Juvenile and Criminal Justice

13. HM Prison Service 1999 Response and action plans. London: HM Prison Service, December

14. Smith R 1984 Women in prison. BMJ 288(6417):630–633

15. Smith R 1999 Prisoners: an end to second class health care? BMJ 318(7189):954–955

16. Reed JL, Lyne M 2000 Inpatient care of mentally ill people in prison: results of a year's programme of semistructured inspections. BMJ 320(7241):1031–1034

17. United Nations 1990 Recommendation of the 8th United Nations congress on the prevention of crime and the treatment of offenders, Cuba. Available at: http://www.asc41.com/undocs.htm (accessed November 2004)

18. Owers A 2003 We should care about our prisons. The Independent, 13 November

19. Lady Stern 2004 Debate on women in prison. Hansard, House of Lords, 28 October, column 1454

21

Pregnant asylum seekers: the dispossessed

The situation I am in makes me to believe that I don't have any value and I'm nothing for ever. Because even the animals from the zoo they treat them nicely. What can I say? Who am I? What can I say? Nothing. What can I do? Nothing. This is how I must live.[1]

Women are very strong. Nine months seems like nine minutes. I try to forget my past.[2]

At any one time there are 13 million refugees worldwide.[3] Most are women and children, the first to be uprooted, and the most vulnerable, wherever disaster strikes or there are human rights violations.

A person who enters the UK seeking asylum must apply at the port of entry or within 3 days of arriving. Even if this is done, an asylum seeker may be detained at any stage of the asylum claim, without having committed any crime, and often without knowing why they are being locked up. Communication is difficult because they are often unable to speak English. No figures are released as to the number of pregnant women and babies in detention, nor about the number who give birth. They become dependent on charity, on friends, or the kindness of strangers. In the first 6 months of 2004, for example, 100 Eritrean women, many of them rape survivors, sought help from the All-African Women's Group, The Black Women's Rape Action Project, Legal Action for Women and Women Against Rape. In May of that year, Amnesty International documented systematic human rights violations in Eritrea and called on the international community to protect refugees from that country. But the Home Office continued to turn down Eritrean women's applications for asylum and would consider them only individually – a slow and tortuous process that often resulted in them being refused asylum.

Families in detention become invisible. There is no time limit on it. 'There are few safeguards against lengthy detention because, unlike almost all other European countries, in the UK there is no statutory time limit on detention and no automatic access to an independent body to review detention'.[4] The Prime Minister, Tony Blair, announced in September 2004 that 1000 more places in detention centres were to be created. A woman can be moved from one detention centre to another without notice. 'They woke me at 7 a.m. and said "In 15 minutes you're going to [another detention centre]". I had no time to say goodbye to anyone. I managed to make two bottles of milk, but the journey was really hard – 8 hours in a van with a baby who had been sick for the 2 days before they moved us. They haven't told me why they moved us'.[5] Another woman, whose baby had been taken from her by deception in an attempt to expel her, said: 'because they came to take my baby, I am worried all the time, whenever I hear keys. I can't sleep at night – a small noise and I'm awake. I walk around at night – just walk, walk'.[6]

> Women seeking asylum may arrive in England having lost everything they value: children, partner, parents, extended family, community, home, job, health, money, possessions, culture ... The special needs of pregnant asylum seekers and their babies have been largely ignored in the context of a support system designed to have a deterrent effect on people seeking to come to the UK.[7]

Pregnant women and new mothers fleeing war, famine, torture and oppression who manage to get to Britain face discrimination, poverty and blatant injustice. It is part of Government policy to show that we are not 'a soft touch'. Until recently (2004), once an asylum seeker's application was refused, any help she had been receiving from Social Services was withdrawn. Now it is up to the local Social Services department to make an 'assessment' and decide whether to provide the woman with housing. Social Services have different policies in different areas. The advice line of the Refugee Council states that any accommodation will be *temporary* and available only while the mother is breastfeeding. If she continues to breastfeed beyond the time they consider reasonable (3 months or so), she will be told to leave the country. If she fails to do this, they take the baby away.

Some women are destitute. They live on the streets and sleep in bus shelters. With no address, a general practitioner (GP) is unlikely to accept them, except for urgent treatment. A hospital clinic may be a distance away. One woman said, 'I walk to the hospital; it takes 2½ hours'.[8] There is a reimbursement scheme, but many are unaware of it and, without cash, could not benefit from it anyway.

These women are often in need of medical care. They may have been in a refugee camp before escaping. Conditions in these camps are poor, and epidemics of disease sweep through them. There may be higher mortality there than in the country from which they have fled. There is often sexual violence, too.[5]

Around the world, 113 million girls and women have experienced ritual genital mutilation.[8] The consequences include pelvic pain, dyspareunia or inability to have intercourse, rectovaginal fistulas, chronic pelvic inflammatory disease, urinary tract infections and scar abscesses. It may be impossible for a pelvic examination to be done and it is very likely that a woman will need a perineal incision before she can give birth.

At the end of May 2004 the Court of Appeal ruled that the ban on asylum seekers from housing and other benefits was illegal and in breach of human rights. They are entitled to support while an asylum claim is pending. A pregnant woman can get support under the National Assistance Act and, once the baby is born, under the Children's Act if she can prove that she is 'in need of care and attention'. But it is not enough for her to be destitute. She has to prove that she has diabetes or is mentally ill, for example. The National Asylum Support Service does not tell asylum seekers about this, and if a woman asks for help from Social Services there is a good chance that she will be turned away. Everything depends on finding a good lawyer.

It is difficult to get legal help. The Home Office have cut Legal Aid, so there is a severe shortage of lawyers willing to take on these cases. Some of the solicitors available are incompetent or corrupt. Women may be asked to pay or to provide sexual services in return for legal representation. If women are not fluent in speaking and writing English, it may be impossible for them to represent themselves.

Even when a mother of small children gets support, the exact amount is discretionary, and far less than under Income Support. It varies from local authority to local authority and social worker to social worker. Some women only get hospital accommodation, but no money. One woman received £25 a week for herself and her baby, but is being subjected to regular questioning by Social Services because she looks well dressed (her clothing is donated by a woman's centre).

Asylum seekers whose applications have been turned down often go into hiding. They avoid anyone who seems to represent authority, and this includes healthcare professionals. They have good reason to do so. The National Conference of The Royal College of Midwives passed a resolution in March 2004 that stated 'Conference calls on Council to challenge any moves by the Government that may result in midwives being required to act as inspectors policing the receipt of benefits and immigration controls'.[9]

GPs are also protesting about rules that require them to vet new patients for their residency status before treating them. The Institute of Healthcare Management states: 'Practice managers and GPs should not be expected to become a hidden arm of the immigration services'.[10]

A GP who works with asylum seekers points out:

> *Failed asylum seekers are not bogus asylum seekers. Of 58,475 decisions on asylum made by the Home Office in 2003–2004, 87% were refused, 21%*

were accepted, leaving 60,000 failed asylum seekers. Although some of these people may not be in need of protection, many certainly are but are unable to establish to a 'reasonable degree of likelihood' that they would suffer persecution if returned to their country ... Each day in my general practice I see people who have been refused asylum who fear being returned home. Frequently this is because they have been imprisoned, tortured, or raped. Sometimes it is because they have witnessed relatives being killed, have been evicted from their homes, or have been beaten because of their politics or sexuality. Many carry no documentary evidence because they fled in fear of their lives, or carry 'only' psychological scars that do not convince decision makers of their suffering ... If a failed asylum seeker is being treated at intervals of 7 days or less then they can 'continue to receive the treatment free of charge until such a time as that person no longer needs such treatment'. This allows a GP to treat for conjunctivitis, but not to provide care for pregnancy, post-traumatic stress disorder, or incontinence.[11]

Another major injustice is the policy of 'dispersal'. The National Asylum Support Service has responsibility to disperse asylum seekers. It allocates them to 'emergency accommodation'. If accepted, they are sent to different parts of the country, often at short notice. A mother of a new baby, for example, was told she must board a bus in 5 days time with any belongings she could carry with her to go either to Glasgow or Birmingham, and she would be told where when in transit. Women land up in places where they have no support network, often not speaking English, isolated and outcast. Midwives and doctors first know that their patients have disappeared when they fail to turn up for antenatal appointments. At least one woman has been dispersed when already in labour. When women are moved to detention centres their children are taken into care. There has been strong criticism of the practice of holding children in 'family rooms' in detention centres. The policy now is to remove the children. Mothers may not know where their children have gone or when they will ever see them again. This happens even to children as young as 18 months old who cannot understand English.

Some women with babies are virtually children themselves. Roma (Gypsy) mothers are arrested for begging on London Underground stations. In Roma culture a girl is adult and may marry at 14 years of age. She breastfeeds her own baby and those of other family members. The Roma consider bottles dirty and unhealthy. She is often arrested with one child of her own and up to three other babies or toddlers. If her parents have been deported to Romania, from which 78% of these girls come, or to another East European country, she has the responsibility to get money to send back to them. When she is picked up by the police she may be kept in custody for some days, Social Services take the babies into care, and if she is accused of theft, the separation may be much longer.

Asylum seekers whose application has been turned down can only survive on charity, or by begging, petty theft or finding a man to protect them (who may turn out to be a pimp). With no money to buy nappies, they use newspaper.

When a woman is destitute, Social Services are likely to take the baby into care because the mother is homeless.

Women have had to leave other children in the country from which they fled. One pregnant woman said: 'I couldn't sleep at night, thinking about the children. I never knew, maybe they are dead, maybe they are alive, maybe something else happened to them, because in Freetown when the rebels took it, they just took off the hands of kids ... I am waiting, because you just have to wait, it's very stressful, because the more you start thinking about it, the more you suffer from the thinking, because when you start thinking it just doesn't stop there, you are thinking wider, wider, wider, so you become stressed'.[1]

Rape is used as a method of torture. Before they have fled their homes many women have been raped. Catherine (not her real name), for example, fled to Britain from Eritrea after all her family were killed and she refused military service. She was imprisoned in a detention centre in Eritrea for 3 years, where she was beaten and raped repeatedly. She was refused asylum in the UK, was pregnant and destitute, and spoke no English. When she gave birth in spring 2004 the midwife noticed vaginal fistulas that may have resulted from rape; she needs reconstructive surgery. Perhaps that physical evidence of torture will enable her to get asylum.

Women who have been raped are often not believed by the authorities unless they can show evidence of physical injury – cigarette burns and scars to the genitals, laceration, or cutting away of the clitoris and labia. But the Medical Foundation for the Victims of Torture explains that 'rape usually presents no physical evidence'.[12]

They often feel ashamed and dirty. A Sri Lankan woman was raped by government forces when 8 months pregnant. She cleans herself and the house over and over again and shows no recognition of her baby's existence. She says she was 'contaminated by what happened to me', and feels that the rapist's semen must have covered her baby.[13]

Many women develop post-traumatic stress disorder and have nightmares and flashbacks to the event. This may be combined with depression and emotional fragmentation. One woman described it this way: 'If a metal is damaged it will show the damage by bending. If china is damaged it will shatter and no longer be as it was before. Even a stone can break if enough force is used. But what happened to me – my body stayed whole on the outside but inside it is so broken and no one can see the damage'.

One effect is that survivors may not be able to recount a coherent story. The principal psychiatrist at the Medical Foundation for the Victims of Torture, Abigail Seltzer, comments: 'Avoidance, patchy memory and impaired concentration may lead to apparent inconsistencies, omissions or lack of detail. This can have serious implications for those seeking asylum, as without an understanding of how affective and cognitive function can be devastated by such a trauma, there is a risk that officials will simply dismiss victims as "faking it".[14] The gynaecologist at the Medical Foundation explains: 'It is extraordinarily difficult to prove this crime beyond all reasonable doubt'.[15]

In UK domestic law rape does not constitute torture unless it is part of 'a consistent course of violence over a period of time'.[16] This is at variance with European law, in which a single act of rape can constitute torture. There are also cases in which asylum has been refused and women deported to countries from which they have fled on the grounds that their age and appearance make it unlikely that they will be raped again. A 52-year-old Sri Lankan woman was deported on the grounds that she was in no danger because 'without wishing to appear unchivalrous, we have to say that there can be no significant risk of rape at her age'.[17]

A woman who bears a child as a result of rape may love her baby and caring for it may be part of the healing process. Or she may find it difficult to bond. Mothers often help each other. When a support network is destroyed it can be emotionally disastrous. An asylum seeker who could not cope with the conflicting feelings she felt for her baby gained great support from another asylum seeker. They cared for their babies together. But the National Asylum Support Service separated the two women, and this mother was left distraught.

The Sixth Report of the Confidential Enquiries into Maternal Deaths in the UK for 2000–2002 noted that Black African women, including asylum seekers and newly arrived refugees, had a mortality rate seven times higher than white women and major problems in accessing maternal health care. It recommended: 'Asylum seekers and refugees are a particularly vulnerable group and services need to respond to their needs. Professional interpreters should be provided for women who do not speak English. The use of family members, including children should be avoided if at all possible'. It went on to say: 'Health professionals who work with disadvantaged clients need to be able to understand a woman's social and cultural background, act as an advocate for women with other colleagues and address their own personal and social prejudices and practice in a reflective manner. All healthcare professionals should consider whether there are unrecognised but inherent racial prejudices within their own organisations, in terms of providing an equal service to all women'.[18]

I believe that in every country where there are large numbers of asylum seekers there needs to be an advocacy service for those who are pregnant and have young children. The training of advocates might be based on the effective system of voluntary advocates that is already well established throughout the UK for mental health patients. In Auckland, New Zealand, I was struck by the effectiveness and warmth of the Advocacy Service at the Women's Hospital that has been run for many years for Maori and Polynesian women, for others who are socially disadvantaged and for members of ethnic minorities. In the UK, at present, any help a woman gets comes from voluntary helpers, sections of the Social Services, and projects such as Sure Start, which focuses on one-to-one care for teenage girls, substance abusers and ethnic minority women. Help is uncoordinated: it is not sufficient to have interpreters when a woman visits an antenatal clinic, for example. She needs someone who understands how the health services work, knows about birth and the terminology used by doctors, and can help her negotiate the kind of care she needs. Asylum seekers often experience intense loneliness and isolation. They need continuing friendship and support from another woman whom they can trust and who understands what they are going through. They need someone who can stand up to powerful institutions and give these women a voice.

References

1. McLeish J 2002 Mothers in exile: maternity experiences of asylum seekers in England. Report. London: Maternity Alliance, March, p 55–56

2. McLeish J 2002 Mothers in exile: maternity experiences of asylum seekers in England. Report. London: Maternity Alliance, March, p 69

3. US Committee for Refugees 2004 World refugee survey 2004. Available at: http://www.refugees.org/wrs04/main.html (accessed November 2004)

4. Maternity Alliance 2001 A crying shame: pregnant asylum seekers and their babies in detention. Bail for immigration detainees. Briefing paper. London: Maternity Alliance, December, p 10. Available at: http://www.maternityalliance.org.uk/ prof_health.htm#4 (accessed November 2004)

5. Adams KM, Gardiner LD, Assefi N 2004 Healthcare challenges from the developing world: post-immigration refugee medicine. BMJ 328(7455):1548–1552

6. McLeish J 2002 Maternity alliance briefing paper. London: Maternity Alliance, March, p 1. Available at: http://www.refugees.org/wrs04/main.html (accessed November 2004)

7. McLeish J 2002 Mothers in exile: maternity experiences of asylum seekers in England. Report. London; Maternity Alliance, March, p 35

8. Toubia N 1999 Caring for women with circumcision: a technical manual for providers. New York: Rainbo

9. Royal College of Midwives 2002 Resolution passed. National Conference, Swansea, June

10. Kmietowicz Z 2004 GPs to check on patients' residency status to stop 'health tourism'. BMJ 328(7450):1217

11. Williams PD 2004 Why failed asylum seekers must not be denied access to the NHS. BMJ 329(7460):298

12. Clarke P 2004 Physical consequences of rape of women. In: Peel M (ed) Rape as a method of torture. London: Medical Foundation for the Care of Victims of Torture, p 133

13. Avigad AJ, Rahimi Z 2004 Impact of rape on the family: physical consequences of rape of women. In: Peel M (ed) Rape as a method of torture. London: Medical Foundation for the Care of Victims of Torture, p 126

14. Seltzer A. Rape and mental health: the psychiatric sequelae of violation as an abuse of human rights. In: Peel M (ed) Rape as a method of torture. London: Medical Foundation for the Care of Victims of Torture, p 107

15. Clarke P 2004 Physical Consequences of rape of women. In: Peel M (ed) Rape as a method of torture. London: Medical Foundation for the Care of Victims of Torture, p 200

16. R.v. Special Adjudicator ex parte Ogochukwu Chigioke Okonkwo [1998] Imm AR 502

17. Mariamma d/o Thevashayam v. The Secretary of State for the Home Department, Immigration Appeal Tribunal, 31 January 2002

18. Lewis G, Drife J 2004 Why Mothers die: confidential enquiry into maternal and child health. Sixth Report. London: RCOG Press, p 10. Executive Summary and Midwifery Summary available at: http://www.cemach.org.uk/publications.htm (accessed November 2004)

22

Changing our birth culture

So where do we go from here? How do we work together to bring about a metamorphosis from the technocratic model of birth to a social model that is more satisfying for everyone? How do we reach out to care for the most vulnerable women and babies in our society?

Redefining the role of the midwife

For midwives to give of their best, to be able to fill a multidimensional role, they need to be free to have a one-to-one relationship with their clients and to make their own clinical judgements. Both the midwife and the mother benefit from continuity in their relationship.

The midwife must be free to take professional responsibility during childbirth, too. However non-interventionist she is, however relaxed, she is not just knitting in the corner. Nor is she intent on writing up her notes while the woman labours alone. She is not down the hallway at the nursing station discussing last night's party; nor staring anxiously at a monitor, ignoring the mother. She does not stand over her patient, snapping out orders like a boxing coach. She gives the woman space and confidence to follow the rhythms of her body. This often means standing back. But at the same time she is alert and observant.

Redefining the identity of the midwife must be linked with knowledge of research taking place internationally that has direct bearing on ways in which women experience birth and early motherhood, and the role of the midwife in creating a facilitating environment for a major life process. The new midwifery is *evidence-based*. That entails being up-to-date with research and being able to evaluate it rigorously. It also means bringing the same critical faculties to randomised controlled trials as to other research evidence, and not treating them as laws engraved in stone.

Searching questions have to be asked, not only about interventions made by obstetricians, but also about all childbirth practices, including those hallowed by time – all the usual admission procedures when a woman enters hospital, frequent vaginal examinations, and confining her to bed or in a room in which the bed is the central object. We need to question also those customary interventions made by midwives, such as asking a woman whether she wants to push. That is like asking 'Do you want to swallow?' Or telling her to push and hold her breath. That is like trying to *teach* someone how to swallow. Midwives must challenge dogma and rigid institutional practices in the light of evidence. This means that leadership has to come from *within* the midwifery service itself, not be superimposed upon it.

When midwives become well informed and question their own practice they move on to the cutting edge of healthcare. A cutting edge is a very uncomfortable place to be. It almost inevitably entails confrontation and conflict with the existing order of large, hierarchical institutions. Institutions change slowly, ponderously. Research has demonstrated that it takes, on average, 15 years from the time the results of randomised controlled trials in obstetrics are published and to a change in hospital practice. That time is bound to be painful.

Midwives need to learn and develop further the science and the art of keeping birth normal. This is not, however, only a matter of intellectual understanding. An important element is acknowledging the vital role of the midwife who has the skills to hold, cradle, massage, nurture and sustain. Giving birth can be, in the deepest and most meaningful sense, a sexual experience. I am not talking about orgasm. I mean vivid, concentrated, satisfying, psycho-physical experience.

This is where midwives have a very important function. For they can liberate women to experience the intense spirituality and exhilaration of birth. To do this, they have to honour and protect the powerful surge of hormone energy that comes when a woman trusts her body and is in an environment in which she can act spontaneously.

The revolution that needs to take place is both at the level of the intellect and in midwives' hearts. The synthesis of thought and feeling, of expert skills, understanding the normal and deviations from the normal, the synthesis of knowledge and sensitivity, will create the midwifery of the future.

Open eyes – exploring minds

In all interaction between midwives, health visitors, doctors and others who care for pregnant women, those in labour and new mothers, it is vital to listen and learn, instead of *telling* and hoping that those at the receiving end are absorbing the teaching.

Learning is at its most effective when it is part of a process of discovery. That is as true for professionals as it is for women having babies. Something can be learned from every single woman. Only then can we enter a relationship with her in which, in an old Quaker phrase, we 'speak to her condition'; only then can we relate to her as a unique human being.

It is often claimed that communication is the answer to problems in the maternity services. Yes, but only up to a point. Handing out leaflets to provide information, offering advice, and screening patients for physical illness, psychological states and social conditions, mentally ticking boxes and filling out forms, amounts to what Mavis Kirkham, Professor of Midwifery at Sheffield, calls 'communication without relationship'.[1] The skills of building relationships and opening our minds so that we learn from each individual, even the most unlikely, lie at the heart of insight and understanding. We need to be there for women, without distancing ourselves, without hesitation.

Analysing our birth culture

Simultaneously, I believe that we need to develop sociological awareness of how professionals and childbearing women see themselves and each other, how power and powerlessness are expressed, how large institutions such as hospitals function, and the ways in which this affects human interaction. The study of birth in its social context is sometimes seen as being about 'ethnicity' – caring for women in minority groups who pose problems for management. To approach the sociology of birth in that way means that we fail to see how the birth culture of which we are a part affects our *own* assumptions and behaviour and those of our colleagues.

There is a good deal of conflict in midwifery at present. A midwife who works for change may be marginalised and feel isolated. If each midwife thinks of herself as a solitary warrior fighting a lonely battle the struggle is bound to be frustrating and exhausting. She tends to perceive each assault as personally directed against her, and blames individuals who themselves are usually slaves of a system that is out of their control. We need to acknowledge that technocratic birth often traps caregivers into being cogs in a machine, just as it directs those being cared for onto a conveyor belt from which they cannot escape. When midwives or patients are bullied or humiliated, for instance, it is not a matter for blame and self-blame, accusation and counter-accusation, so much as understanding how power and subjugation operate in hierarchical institutions. It is the *system* that needs changing.

Midwives and others in the health services need to work together to humanise the system. The challenge is to explore the dynamics of social interaction in our technocratic birth culture and work out what should be changed, and how this can be done. This is not just a matter of acquiring information. Knowledge has to be *used*. Learning needs to be incorporated in practice. Plutarch said: 'A mind is a fire to be kindled, not a vessel to be filled'. The fire in our minds needs to be expressed in *action* at the level of the personal and the political. This action will change our birth culture. Midwives can become better carers, and more effective researchers, activists and advocates for women.

References

1.   Kirkham M 2004 Informed choice in maternity care. New York: Palgrave McMillan

Reflections

Chapters 1–3

After reading the last three chapters it may help you consider the information and ideas I put forward to answer these questions:

1. How can control of the birth environment affect labour?
2. Who has control of the birth place and the interaction of people in it in traditional, social childbirth?
3. Who controls the birth place in contemporary technocratic birth?

Chapters 4–6

When you have read these three chapters here is a project:

1. Collect together visual images and references in words to birth and breastfeeding from newspapers, magazines and TV.
2. What do they tell us about social perception of these activities?

Language of birth, touch and its meaning

Analyse the language used in an obstetric textbook.

1. How are women's bodies represented?
2. What kinds of touch are described?

Caesarean epidemic, court-ordered caesareans

Two or three women are discussing the kind of birth they want. There is one who hopes for an elective caesarean, another who hopes for a vaginal birth, and perhaps there is another who is very uncertain what she wants. Write up the discussion as if it were a script for a scene in a play.

Birth plans

Ask a woman – several if you can – who has had a previous experience of birth to write a birth plan for her next birth.

1. What does it teach you about the woman, her previous birth experience, and how her caregivers can relate to her in the coming birth? Discuss this with her.

Home birth, waterbirth, birth dance

Imagine that you are a woman expecting your first baby and are seeking information about the choices available. Go to a general practitioner's clinic and collect any leaflets on display, including any you can find that deal with the topics of home birth, waterbirth and movement in childbirth. How are these choices presented?

If you are unable to obtain information, or the information you get is sketchy, write a leaflet yourself that might be useful for pregnant women exploring their options.

What's happening to midwives?

Explore the role of midwives in several countries through a web search. Write up your findings.

Suggestions of websites you might want to look at include: http://www.birth.hu and http://www.parteras.org

Doulas, fathers, children at birth

Consider the different people who may be at a birth and why. Talk to some individuals who attended a birth and discover what their experience was.

Silence is collusion, mothers behind bars, pregnant asylum seekers

Discuss issues about power and powerlessness and conditions for pregnant women and mothers of young children who are abused, in UK prisons, or seeking asylum. Do a web search to get up-to-date information.

Suggestions for websites you can go into are: http://www.prisonreformtrust.org.uk and http:www.hmprisonservice.gov.uk

Birth in our culture

1. What would you change about birth in our culture?
2. How would you start doing this?

Useful websites and addresses

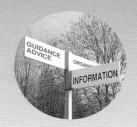

Giving birth

UK

Active Birth Centre
Tel: 020 72816760
http://www.activebirthcentre.com

Cochrane Database
http://www.thecochranelibrary.com

Sheila Kitzinger
Tel: 01865 300266
E-mail: sheila@sheilakitzinger.com
http://www.sheilakitzinger.com

Maternity Alliance
Tel: 020 7490 7638
http://www.maternityalliance.org.uk

National Childbirth Trust (NCT)
Tel: 08 70 444 8707
http://www.nctpregnancyandbabycare.com

Royal College of Obstetricians and Gynaecologists
Tel: 020 7772 6200
http://www.rcog.org.uk

USA

Bradley Method: American Academy of Husband-Coached Childbirth
Tel: 800-4-A-BIRTH or 800 423 2397
http://www.bradleybirth.com

International Childbirth Education Association (ICEA)
Tel: 800 368 4404
http://www.icea.org

Lamaze International (US)
Tel: 202 367 1128
Toll-Free: 800 368 4404
http://www.lamaze-childbirth.com

National Association of Childbearing Centers
Tel: 215 234 8068
E-mail: ReachNACC@BirthCenters.org
http://www.birthcenters.org

Home birth

UK

Birth Choice UK
http://www.birthchoiceuk.com

Home Birth Reference Site
http://www.homebirth.org.uk

USA

American College of Home Obstetrics
Tel: 847 455 2030

Informed Homebirth and Informed Parenting
Tel: 616 961 6923

Support

UK

Birth Crisis
Tel: 01865 300266
E-mail: birthcrisis@sheilakitzinger.com
http://www.sheilakitzinger.com/
    Birth %20Crisis.htm
Helps those who are distressed after birth.

Brazelton Centre in Great Britain
E-mail: info@brazelton.co.uk
http://www.brazelton.co.uk
Understanding newborn behaviour and supporting early parent–infant relationships.

Contact a Family
Tel: 0808 808 3555
http://www.cafamily.org.uk
Helps parents of disabled children get in touch with other families.

Gingerbread
Tel: 0800 018 4318
http://www.gingerbread.co.uk
Support group for single parents.

Mothers over 40
http://www.mothersover40.com

Parentline
Tel: 0808 800 2222
http://www.parentline.co.uk

Stillbirth and Neonatal Death Society
Tel: 020 74367940
http://www.uk-sands.org

Maternity care

Baby Lifeline
Empathy Enterprise Building,
    Bramston Crescent, Tile Hill,
    Coventry CV4 9SW
Tel: 0845 6581059 (local rate)
    024 7642 2135
E-mail: info@babylifeline.org.uk
http://www.babylifeline.org.uk

USA

Disability, Pregnancy and Parenthood International
Auburn Press, 9954 South Walnut
    Terrace, No. 201, Palos Hills,
    IL 60465

FertilityPlus
http://www.fertilityplus.org/faq/
    miscarriage/resources.html
Information on support groups, medical information, and books about miscarriage.

Gay & Lesbian Parents Coalition International
Tel: 202 583 8029

Waterbirth

UK

Active Birth Centre
Tel: 020 72816760
http://www.activebirthcentre.com

UK Aquanatal Register
Tel: 01628 661961
http://www.aquanatal.co.uk

Edgware Birth Centre
Tel: 020 87326777
http://www.birthcentre.co.uk

National Childbirth Trust
Tel: 0870 4448707
http://www.nct-online.org

Primal Health Research Centre
E-mail: modent@aol.com
http://www.birthworks.org/primalhealth

USA

Global Maternal/Child Health
Association, Inc.
Tel: 503 673 0026
E-mail: info@waterbirth.org
http://www.waterbirth.org

Portable pool hire companies

UK

Active Birth Pools
Tel: 020 72721311
http://www.activebirthpools.com

Active Birth Centre
Tel: 020 72816760
http://www.activebirthcentre.com

Birth-Pool-in-a-Box
Tel: 0870 7201207
http://www.birthpoolinabox.co.uk

Birth Works
Tel: 01227 830880
http://www.birthworks.co.uk

BubbaTubs
Tel: 01992 302449
http://www.bubbatubs.com

Gentle Water
Tel: 01273 474927
http://www.gentlewater.co.uk

The Good Birth Company
Tel: 0800 0350514
http://www.thegoodbirth.co.uk

Splashdown Water Birth
Services Ltd
Tel: 0870 444 4403
http://www.splashdown.org.uk

USA

Global Maternal/Child Health
Association, Inc.
Tel: 503 673 0026
E-mail: info@waterbirth.org
http://www.waterbirth.org

Breastfeeding

World Alliance for Breastfeeding
Action
http://www.waba.org.my

UK

Association of Breastfeeding
Mothers
Tel: 020 7813 1481
http://www.abm.me.uk

Breastfeeding Network
Tel: 0870 900 8787
http://www.breastfeedingnetwork.org.uk

La Leche League
Tel: 020 7242 1278
http://www.laleche.org.uk

National Childbirth Trust
Tel: 0870 4448707
http://www.nctpregnancyandbabycare.
com

USA

International Lactation Consultants
Association (ILCA)
Tel: 919 787 5181
E-mail: ilca@erols.com
http://www.ilca.org

La Leche League International
Tel: 800 525 3243 (Breastfeeding
Helpline)
http://www.lalecheleague.org

Australia

Breastfeeding Mothers of Australia
http://www.breastfeeding.asn.au

Comprehensive breastfeeding site
http://www.breastfeeding.com

Preterm babies

UK

Bliss the Premature Baby Charity
Tel: 0500 618140
http://www.bliss.org.uk

USA

Kangaroo Care
http://www.geocities.com/roopage
*A site on the benefits of 'kangaroo care',
and skin-to-skin contact, for pre-term
babies.*

Premature Baby – Premature Child
http://www.prematurity.org

Caesareans

USA

International Cesarean Awareness
Network
http://www.ican-online.org

Midwives

UK

Albany Midwives Practice
Tel: 020 75254995
E-mail: albanymidwives@ukonline.co.uk

ARM (Association of Radical Midwives)
Tel: 0121 444 2257
http://www.radmid.demon.co.uk

Independent Midwives Association
Tel: 01483 821104
E-mail: c.f.winter@city.ac.uk
http://www.independentmidwives.org.uk

MIDIRS (Midwives Information & Resource Service)
Tel: 0117 9251791
      0800 581009 (UK only)
http://www.midirs.org

Nursing and Midwifery Council
Tel: 020 7637 7181
http://www.nmc-uk.org

Royal College of Midwives
Tel: 020 73123535
E-mail: info@rcm.org.uk
http://www.rcm.org.uk

USA

American College of Nurse Midwives (ACNM)
Tel: 202 728 9868
E-mail: info@acnm.org
http://www.acnm.org

Citizens for Midwifery
http://www.cfmidwifery.org

Coalition to Improve Maternity Services (CIMS)
Tel: 202 478 6138

Midwives Alliance of North America (MANA)
Tel: 888 923 6262
http://www.mana.org

Midwifery Information
http://www.midwifeinfo.com

Doulas

UK

Doula UK
PO Box 26678, London N14 4WB
Tel: 0871 433 3101
E-mail: info@doula.org.uk
http://www.doula.org.uk

USA

BirthPartners.Com LLC
0029 Crystal Cove, PO Box 2632,
      Dillon, CO 80435
Tel: 970 262 6692
Cell: 970 389 3115
E-mail: Montane@BirthPartners.com
http://www.birthpartners.com

Doulas of North America (DONA)
Tel (Toll-Free): 888 788-DONA
E-mail: doula@DONA.org
http://www.DONA.org

Complementary therapies

UK

Aromatherapy Consortium
Tel: 0870 774 3477
http://www.aromatherapy-regulation.org.uk

Association of Qualified Curative Hypnotherapists
Tel: 0121 6931223
http://www.aqch.org

British Acupuncture Council
Tel: 020 8735 0400
http://www.acupuncture.org.uk

British Society of Medical and Dental Hypnotists
Tel: 07000 560309
http://www.bsmdh.com

Northern College of Acupuncture
Tel: 01904 343305
http://www.chinese-medicine.co.uk

British Homeopathic Association
Tel: 0870 4443950
http://www.trusthomeopathy.org

British Institute of Homeopathy
Tel: 01784 440467
http://www.britinsthom.com

British Reflexology Association
Tel: 01886 821207
http://www.britreflex.co.uk

General Osteopathic Council
Tel: 020 73576655
http://www.osteopathy.org.uk

International Federation of Reflexologists
Tel: 020 86459134
http://www.reflexology-ifr.com

National Council for Hypnotherapy
Tel: 0800 9520545
http://www.hypnotherapists.org.uk

National Institute of Medical Herbalists
Tel: 44 (0)1392 426022
http://www.nimh.org.uk

Society of Teachers of the Alexander Technique
Tel: 0845 2307828
http://www.stat.org.uk

Shiatsu for Midwives
Tel: 0117 9632306
http://www.wellmother.org

Birth Light
http://www.birthlight.com
Information on yoga, aqua yoga and baby yoga classes.

British Wheel of Yoga
Tel: 01529 306851
http://www.bwy.org.uk

USA

American Association of Naturopathic Physicians
Tel: 206 298 0126
http://www.naturopathic.org

American Chiropractic Association
Tel: 703 276 8800
E-mail: memberinfo@amerchiro.org

American Holistic Health Association
Tel: 714 779 6152
E-mail: ahha@healthy.net
http://www.ahha.org

American Holistic Medical Association
Tel: 703 556 9245
http://www.holisticmedicine.org

National Acupuncture and Oriental Medicine Alliance
Tel: 253 851 6896
http://www.acuall.org

National Certification Commission for Acupuncture and Oriental Medicine
Tel: 703 548 9004

The National Institute of Ayurvedic Medicine
Tel: 888 246 NIAM
http://www.niam.com

North American Society of Homeopaths (NASH)
Tel: 206 720 7000
http://www.homeopathy.org

The National Center for Complementary and Alternative Medicine (NCCAM)
Tel: 888 644 6226
http://nccam.nih.gov

The Reflexology Association of America
4012 S. Rainbow Boulevard, Box K585, Las Vegas, NV 89103-2059
http://www.reflexology-usa.org

Health

UK

Antenatal Results and Choices (ARC)
Tel: 020 7631 0285
http://www.arc-uk.org

Cochrane Database
http://www.thecochranelibrary.com

Department of Health
Tel: 020 72104580
http://www.doh.gov.uk

Diabetes UK
Tel: 020 74241030
http://www.diabetes.org.uk

Eating for Pregnancy Helpline
Tel: 0845 1303646
E-mail: pregnancy.nutrition @sheffield.ac.uk

Medical Research Council
Tel: 020 7636 5422
http://www.mrc.ac.uk

NHS Direct
Tel: 0845 4647
http://www.nhsdirect.nhs.uk

Royal College of General Practitioners
Tel: 020 7581 3232
E-mail: info@rcgp.org.uk
http://www.rcgp.org.uk

Royal College of Paediatrics & Child Health
Tel: 020 7307 5600
http://www.rcpch.ac.uk

Royal Society of Medicine
Tel: 0207290 2900
http://www.rsm.ac.uk

USA

Association of Prenatal and Perinatal Psychology and Health (APPPAH)
Tel: 707 857 4041
E-mail: apppah@aol.com
http://www.birthpsychology.com

Violence

UK

Action for Victims of Medical
Accidents
Tel: 0845 123 2352
E-mail: admin@avma.org.uk
http://www.avma.org.uk

National Domestic Violence
Helpline
Tel: 08457 023468
    0808 2000 247
E-mail: info@womansaid.org.uk
http://www.womansaid.org.uk

Refuge
Tel: 0808 2000247
http://www.refuge.org.uk

Samaritans
Tel: 08457 909090
http://www.samaritans.org.uk

Shelterline
Tel: 0808 8004444
http://england.shelter.org.uk

Women Against Rape and Black
Women's Rape Action Project
Tel: 020 7482 2496
http://www.womenagainstrape.net

Women's Refuge
Tel:0800 735 6836
E-mail: jerseyrefugeoutreach
    @jerseymail.co.uk

Pregnant asylum seekers

UK

Amnesty International
Tel: 020 7814 6200
http://www.amnesty.org

Bail for Immigration Detainees
Tel: 020 7247 3590
http://www.biduk.org

London Asylum Support Group
http://www.asylumsupport.info

Medical Foundation for the Care
of Victims of Torture
Tel: 020 7697 7777
http://www.torturecare.org.uk

Physicians for Human Rights
Tel: 01382 200 794
http://www.dundee.ac.uk/med&-
    humanrights/SSM/phr/home.html

Refugee Council
Tel: 020 7346 6700
http://www.refugeecouncil.org.uk

USA

US Committee for Refugees
http://www.refugees.org

Pregnant women and mothers in prison

UK

Birth Companions
http://www.birthcompanions.org.uk

Howard League for Penal Reform
Tel: 020 7249 7373
E-mail: info@howardleague.org
http://www.howardleague.org

Prison Reform Trust
Tel: 020 7251 5070
E-mail: prt@prisonreformtrust.org.uk
http://www.prisonreformtrust.org.uk

Prison Service, Women's Policy Group
http://www.hmprisonservice.gov.uk

Changing the birth culture

UK

Active Birth Centre
Tel: 020 72816760
http://www.activebirthcentre.com

AIMS (Association for Improvements in the Maternity Services)
Tel: 0870 765 1453
E-mail: info@aims.org.uk
http://www.aims.org.uk

Sheila Kitzinger
Tel: 01865 300266
E-mail: sheila@sheilakitzinger.com
http://www.sheilakitzinger.com

Maternity Alliance
Tel: 020 7490 7638
http://www.maternityalliance.org.uk

National Childbirth Trust (NCT)
Tel: 0870 444 8707
http://www.nctpregnancyandbabycare.
 com

USA

Citizens for Midwifery
http://www.cfmidwifery.org

Index